MOVE!

How Women Can Achieve Athletic Goals
At Any Age

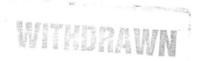
By Catharine Utzschneider, Ed.D.

D1501737

Cedar Crest Books

www.cedarcrestbooks.com

MOVE!
How Women Can Achieve Athletic Goals
At Any Age
by Catharine Utzschneider, Ed.D.
Copyright © 2011 Catharine Utzschneider
ALL RIGHTS RESERVED

First Printing – October 2011
ISBN: 978-0-910291-12-5

Book Design: Kim Davies Designs
Ink line drawing (p. 5): Coreen Steinbach
www.runningart.com

"*MOVE!* captures the needs and desires of all women who want to improve, make changes, and succeed. Cathy has supplied the secret on how to do it. Amazing!"

- *Alison Foley, Head Women's Soccer Coach, Boston College*

"Even if you have a disability or were never an athlete, you can use *MOVE!* for any physical goal. I achieved walking and biking goals I never expected."

- *Nancy Schuder, recreational walker, biker*

"I have experienced first hand the benefits of *MOVE!* for athletics and beyond and have become a huge believer in her goal setting and buddy systems. Knowing you are accountable to someone beside yourself, who is also your cheerleader and will listen when the frustration hits is comforting and helps you to keep MOVING towards your goals."

- *Carmel Papworth-Barnum, World Masters Athletics Track and Field Medalist, Founder www.women-running-together.com*

"*MOVE!* has shown me that most limits are self-imposed. You have no idea what you can achieve so dare to dream and you may surprise yourself."

- *Leni Webber, Recreational runner to national masters champion*

"Cathy changed my life. As a member of the world champion U.S. Lacrosse team and now a graduate student and coach, I have at times felt overwhelmed with lofty goals and the *MOVE!* method gave me an incredible way to break down my ultimate goal into smaller steps and set forth a manageable plan. She has also helped me manage the emotional and mental aspect of the vision and goal I have set for myself, a plan that keeps me on track daily, monthly, and yearly until it is time to compete again."

- Acacia L. Walker, Associate Head Coach, Boston College Women's Lacrosse 10 x Member, World Champion US Lacrosse Team CEO/ Founder, Acacia's Lacrosse

"Cathy is an outstanding coach who understands how to motivate athletes to achieve beyond their own perceived abilities With her as a coach, I set two world records for the mile and a US record for the 3000 meters in the 70 + age group."

- Mary Harada, 4-time Masters World Record Holder, President, Liberty Athletic Club

"Inspiring! Cathy has developed a powerful goal setting method for all athletes, beginners to advanced."

- Dr. Steve Victorson, Founder, Swymfit Strength & Conditioning Coach, U.S. Ski Team 1987-1991

"*MOVE!* speaks to the power of the human spirit. Whether you're young or old, male or female, if you're determined to change yourself for the better, this book will resonate with you!"

- Joe Malloy, National Triathlon Team

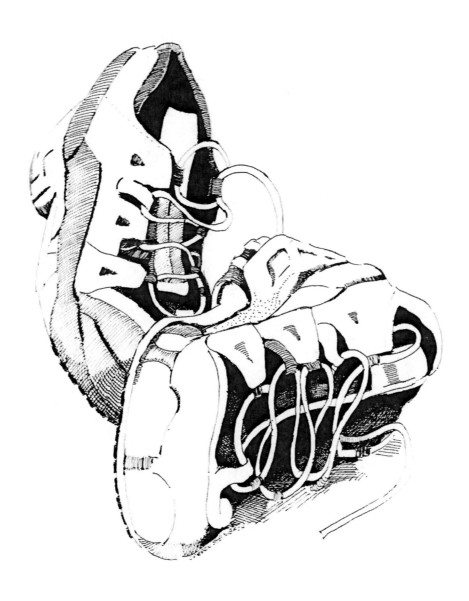

Dedication

This book is dedicated to my family –
Rob, Will, and Annie Utzschneider and to my parents,
Klemens and Elizabeth von Klemperer.

MOVE!

How Women Can Achieve Athletic Goals
At Any Age

Contents

Medical Disclaimer

Always consult your physician before beginning any exercise program. The information herein is not intended to diagnose or treat any medical condition or to replace your healthcare professional. Consult with your healthcare professional to design an appropriate exercise prescription or exercise program.

Your health is your responsibility. Your use of the information contained herein is your choice and will be at your own risk. You as Reader agree that neither the Author nor the Publisher assume any liability for the use or misuse of information contained in this book. You also agree that the information contained herein is provided as is, with no warranties and may not be complete or correct.

The Author and Publisher are not responsible for the content, quality, or accuracy of any book or website referenced or recommended. The reader acknowledges and accepts that the Author and Publisher are not responsible for any information found, referenced and/or recommended in this book such as websites, individuals, organizations and/or other books, nor are they liable to the reader or anyone referenced or quoted herein for any inaccurate, defamatory, offensive, or illegal materials, and the Reader also understands that the risk of injury from viewing, hearing, downloading, or storing such materials rests entirely with the Reader. It is the responsibility of the Reader to evaluate the content, quality, and accuracy of materials or information obtained from other sources.

Not all exercise programs are suitable for everyone, and this or any other program may result in injury. Any user of the information herein assumes the risk of injury resulting from performance of any of the exercises.

Neither the Publisher nor anyone else involved in creating, producing or delivering this book assumes any liability or responsibility for the accuracy, completeness, or usefulness of any information provided (in printed, web or CD format), nor shall they be liable for any direct, indirect, incidental, special, consequential or punitive damages arising out of the use of such information.

The Author and Publisher make no representations or warranties with respect to any exercises, treatment, action, or application of medication or exercises by any person following the information offered or provided within. The Author and Publisher will not be liable for any direct, indirect, consequential, special, exemplary, or other damages arising therefrom.

Acknowledgements

The following people have helped me create this book: Jane Forsyth, who has always believed in me; Father James Woods, Dean of the Woods College of Advancing Studies at Boston College, who invited me to teach and encouraged me to write; Linda Ruth Spitzfaden, who introduced me to my publisher, David Rottenberg, who helped bring the book to life; Jenny Toolin McAuliffe, my superb editor who unquestionably made this a better book; Nancy Schuder and Sue Gustafson who spent weeks reading early rough drafts; Joe Maloy, who spent hours on the forms; Lesley Welch Lehane, whose thoughtful conversation during our runs and walks made my ideas clearer; Zola Budd, who believed in *MOVE!*; Mary Harada, whose athletic performance inspires; Carmel Papworth-Barnum, whose hours of talks drove home the important point of balancing running with other pursuits in life; Randy Sturgeon, who published my articles in National Masters News and connected me with some of the world's best runners; Coreen Steinbach, who contributed her ink line drawing of the sneakers; all the athletes and members of the Liberty Athletic Club who allowed me to coach them; all the women who shared their stories here; and, of course, my family – and, particularly, my husband, Rob.

Foreword

When I started reading the book, I was captivated. The simplicity of the *MOVE!* method is so easy to comprehend and apply, not only in running or in another sport, but in your daily life as well. Cathy understands the perspective and priorities as well as the battles and commitments of being a woman and uses it to apply *MOVE!* to every aspect of our lives.

MOVE! is a practical way to realize your dreams and goals. How many of us have watched a race on television and thought, "I want to do it one day"? Well, with *MOVE!* there are no more excuses. Just MOVE and do it! I like the practicality of the book and the way it visualizes your goals. By keeping logbooks and writing down your training and goals, the level of commitment increases.

MOVE! provides guidelines of how to achieve your goals. It is not just a "how to achieve" book, but it helps you step by step in the whole process, including other commitments like family, friends and work. What I like most about *MOVE!* is the way it approaches setbacks. I have always learned much more from setbacks than from any of my achievements. Setbacks are opportunities to learn. They keep your life in balance. You just need to approach setbacks from a different perspective and allow them to give meaning in your life, as Cathy appropriately shows.

MOVE! is a method you can use not just for your athletic goals – but for all kinds of goals as well. As a mom, you can use it with your kids if you want to teach them. My son wants to learn tennis and my daughter wants to improve her running. I can use the *MOVE!* method to help teach both of them.

Finally, I am looking forward to using the *MOVE!* method myself. I've been planning on doing the Ironman Triathlon next year and had many doubts about if, how, when and can I? After reading Cathy's book, I have the confidence to know that it is possible to realize my goal. (I am not a good swimmer....I swim like a rock.). If you read on, you'll understand that I'll be smiling with a "beginner's mind".

Zola Budd

Two-time World Cross Country Champion
Three-time mom

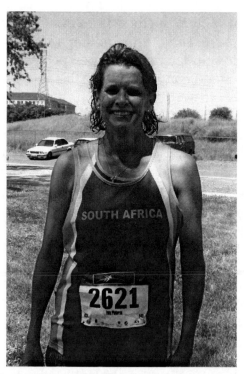

Zola Budd at the 2011 World Masters Athletics Championships.

Preface

As Cathy's coach, training partner, friend, and colleague, I have known about *MOVE!* ever since I met Cathy 14 years ago and I am convinced of the power of *MOVE!*'s message.

Cathy is the perfect person to write this unique book. She is a devoted coach and successful elite masters runner who has a healthy perspective on, and interest in, balancing athletics with the rest of life – family, friends, and career. Cathy started running at 40 and soon established herself as a world-class masters runner. She has served as president of the Liberty Athletic Club, one of the oldest all-female women's running clubs in the country. For the past 20 years, she has coached individuals as well as clubs, including Liberty. As a mother, she is very involved in her children's lives, including having coached her daughter's soccer team for six years.

The message of *MOVE!* is powerful for women wanting to achieve in any sport at any level or ability. As a competitor, teacher and coach myself, I believe strongly in trying to reach your physical potential and know that the *MOVE!* method is valuable in all three endeavors. Through my teaching of children in special education, I have observed first-hand the challenges of learning with disabilities. I have created many games with my students involving *MOVE!* that they find not only fun but also motivating.

I know personally that achieving athletic goals has an amazing impact on the rest of life. No matter who you are or at what stage of life you begin, the *MOVE!* method can help you achieve incredible success in athletics as well as in your professional and personal life.

Lesley Lehane
M.Ed. Special Education
Team USA World Cross Country Champion
Two-time USA National Cross Country Champion
Current World and Former U.S. Record Holder
Three-time mom

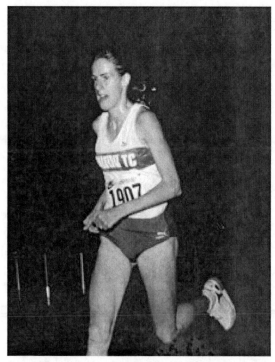

Lesley Lehane racing the 5K indoors.

MOVE!

How Women Can Achieve Athletic Goals
At Any Age

Introduction

"We do not have to become heroes overnight. Just a step at a time, meeting each thing that comes up, seeing it not as dreadful as it appears, discovering that we have the strength to stare it down…. The thing always to remember is that you must do the thing you think you cannot do."
— Eleanor Roosevelt

Think outside your box. Live a longer, stronger life.

It is never too late to take on an athletic goal.

MOVE! (Motivate, Organize, Visualize, Excel) can get you there.

MOVE! is a method of structured goal setting and achievement for every woman.

It has worked for others. **It will work for you.**

Sometimes it's worth changing our routines and beliefs – challenging our habits, the way we live. Why not consider a new perspective, think "outside the box", embrace change and live more fully? Why not create a future we haven't yet imagined?

This book has a simple, straightforward two-part message:

1) No matter what your age is or who you are – whether you've been a lifelong couch potato or a world champion: it is <u>never</u> too late or too hard to design and achieve a new athletic goal that can get you to peak fitness.
2) Achieving that goal can improve your whole life: your career, your relationships, your hobbies, your world.

Sound overpromising? This book presents *MOVE!*, a simple, flexible method that shows you how to achieve athletic – as well as personal and professional goals – and how to enjoy the process along the way.

I know that, regardless of

• whether you are 20, 30, 50, 70 or even 80,
• whether you are a former elite athlete or someone who's never thought of taking on an athletic goal,
• how fit you are,
• any disability you have (arthritis, a chronic illness, even cancer), or
• how chaotic or dull your life is,

MOVE! can help you identify, plan, and achieve a new athletic goal. *MOVE!* can help you gain control of life's responsibilities. It can help you actually *look forward to aging*. It can help you make new friends. The *MOVE!* method of setting and achieving athletic goals has even been used successfully to achieve professional and personal goals. But it all begins with an athletic goal.

A former student of mine who describes herself as "not athletic" gave her perspective on the *MOVE!* method. "The concepts and facts will give you hope," Assistant Dining Service

Manager at Boston College Donna Coleman said. "It's never too late to take on an athletic goal – just knowing about athletic goals is inspiring – and you can begin with something as small as walking for five minutes a day. Hope is important," she said. "That's the carrot. It gives you a little start that you can always remember, something that keeps you positive. My mother who's 72 can do it."

Why Take On An Athletic Goal?

Live a longer, stronger life. Who doesn't want to live a longer, stronger life – one with peaks you never thought possible? Several studies have shown that exercise can add from one to as many as three to four years, as well as higher quality years, to our lives. A study of 16,936 Harvard University alumni found that exercise as simple as walking and stair climbing relates inversely to total mortality (mainly to death due to cardiovascular and respiratory causes).[1]

Another study, based on four decades of data on 4,121 people, confirmed the value of physical activity and particularly of high physical activity in terms of lengthening the lifespan and staving off cardiovascular disease.[2] The study, which divided subjects into three groups of low, medium, and high activity, found that life expectancies at age 50 for the medium and high activity groups were 1.5 and 3.5 years longer respectively than life expectancy for the low activity group. The potential of the aging athlete is not yet known and older athletes are performing better than ever.

---

1. Ralph S. Paffenbarger, Jr., Robert Hyde, Alvin L. Wing, & Chung-cheng Hsieh, "Physical Activity, All-Cause Mortality, and Longevity of College Alumni," The New England Journal of Medicine 314 (1986), 605-613.

2. Oscar H. Franco, Chris de Laet, Anna Peeters, Jacqueline Jonker, Johan Mackenbach, & Wilma Nusselder, "Effects of Physical Activity on Life Expectancy With Cardiovascular Disease", Archives of Internal Medicine 165 (2005), 2355-2360.

Setting achievable athletic goals provides motivation both to exercise and to be our best – our strongest, fastest, and most flexible selves – and helps us live longer, more productive lives.

Surprise yourself beyond your physical prime. Exercise is clearly important not only in keeping our bodies from aging too quickly but also in maximizing our physical potential. Generally, "sarcopenia," or loss of muscle, appears after the age of 40 and accelerates after the age of approximately 75. Physical inactivity causes an average muscle loss of five to seven pounds per decade. But if you exercise, muscle loss will be minimized. As of 2010, Olga Kotelko – who is in her early nineties and still competing in track and field – regularly performed three sets of ten push-ups and three sets of 25 sit-ups. The point? No matter what your age, your physical potential is probably greater than you know and it is never too late to take on an athletic goal, maximize your potential, and reap the benefits.

Running is one sport that confirms ongoing human potential as clearly as any. There is little equipment (other than sneakers) that complicates the calculation of human performance and the clock delivers impartial, objective results. The fact that more and more adults are testing their potential as runners gives scientists plenty of fodder for experiments and conclusions.

Older runners are starting in droves. Today, more records are broken by "masters" runners – those over 40 – than ever. At 50, elite masters runner Carmen Troncoso ran a mile in 5:15 and also set a world age-group record in the 3 kilometer distance in 10:10 and, then, at 51, ran the 3 kilometer in 10:06. It was possible for nonagenarian track and field star Olga Kotelko, to *start* playing softball at 65, and then track and field at 77, and to set dozens of world records in her age group in the interim. Of course world champions are rare birds....but who doesn't feel like a champion after having trained for and reached a goal, any goal, that's represented a challenge?

So, What Is *MOVE!*?

A highly effective method of goal achievement. *MOVE!* stands for Motivate, Organize, Visualize, and Excel. It is a straightforward method of goal setting and achievement for all women. It works – and it's deeply rewarding for those who follow it. It is a method of structured goal setting and guidance to achieve any athletic goal.

This book will take you through both the practical steps and the basic principles to keep in mind to achieve your athletic goal. I will talk more in depth about *MOVE!* in later chapters but, briefly, it's a method I developed over 20 years of coaching, competing, teaching, researching, and writing which involves preparing for, setting, managing, and assessing your athletic goals. The key is to set short-term goals that can point you to long-term goals. It is based on theories of motivation, learning, support, and excellence. Like any process that develops over years, this one has been tweaked, modified, and adapted through my own successes and failures as a competitive athlete as well as of those experienced and inexperienced athletes whom I have coached over the years.

MOVE! has been helping women from recent college graduates to grandmothers reach not just physical goals (they're in the best shape of their lives) but goals in all areas of life. It is a method of simple forms and action steps that were designed for athletic goals but can be tailored to all aspects of life. It's fun and it's easy to follow. The method encourages you to view challenges as opportunities and negatives as positives and how to deal appropriately with life's inevitable setbacks.

Developed from personal experience. I developed the *MOVE!* method when I had an athletic goal in my late twenties and I found something missing. A friend and I wanted to enter New England tennis doubles tournaments and make it through at least a few rounds. We were both working full-time and wanted to be strategic about what strokes to work on, when to practice, and when to play tournaments. We had to find out where and when the tournaments were, and we had to consider everything – training, practice, travel, match play – within the context of our professional and personal lives.

We wanted advice on technique and strategy as well as helpful fitness training but with careers and households to manage, we also wanted someone to integrate our athletic goal into our lives as a whole – someone to help us think about the big picture. We wanted someone to know when we had time to practice, someone with whom to discuss training plans, someone to help construct reasonable short-term goals, and someone to help us figure out strategies to overcome the inevitable hurdles that may be physical, mental, or logistical. We wanted help developing a vision and someone to keep an objective view of what we were doing – someone who might say a particular goal was too aggressive given the time period we chose or given the other limitations in our personal lives.

We approached the tennis pros for help. Ultimately, they said they didn't have the time. They were paid to teach on the courts and didn't have time for off-court coaching. We asked the personal trainers to do the same and found they didn't know much about tennis and didn't show much interest in the other obligations we were juggling.

What were we to do? Give up? You kiddin'?

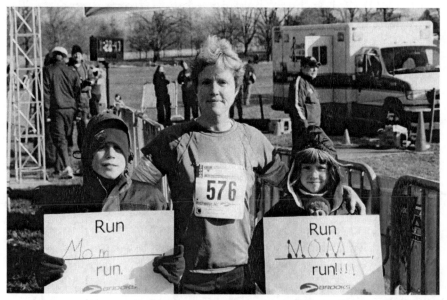

Will, Annie, and I at the national club cross country championships.

We began by being each other's encouragement and creating our own rudimentary forms. We had one for our short-term goal and we kept a daily training log. We met once a week to see whether we were on track. We still took tennis lessons and worked out in the gym but now had an overall strategy that was critical to our success. We won the tournament that year (there were just three rounds).

A few years later, I started a coaching practice based on what I had learned personally about goal setting and training and, over the years, I have developed that into what I call the *MOVE!* method. I have applied it successfully over and over with my clients – elite runners to first-time athletes. It works for them. It has worked for me. I know it will work for you.

PART I

The Theory

The Case For Athletic Goals

*"Find something that you're really interested
in doing in your life. Pursue it, set goals,
and commit yourself to excellence."*
- Chris Evert

Athletic goals help you live longer and stronger.

Specific goals motivate more than a simple fitness routine.

*In addition to better fitness, achieving your athletic goal provides
you with confidence, balance, focus, control and freedom in your
life.*

*Goals can be any improvement over your current level of fitness
in any activity, from walking to hiking to triathlons. You decide.*

*Goals can take anywhere from six weeks to several years. You
decide.*

The Need For Structure

Life for many of us can feel like an overwhelming juggling act. Our lives are complicated and busy and sometimes we can feel as if our lives are like a book with endless words – no sentences, paragraphs, and chapters, with no order and punctuation. Basically, we need structure to progress, not just drift. Without it, time evaporates behind us. We want to meet life challenges to organize the weeks and months and years ahead into a meaningful pattern that captures our individual interests and values, whatever they are. We want a sense of control, balance, strength, mastery and optimism. We want a sense of direction, of going somewhere.

We live in a go-go-go culture. It's a challenge to feel "grounded", to feel that you're moving in a positive direction, whatever that direction may be. Obstacles and distractions abound. They are like weeds. They're everywhere and they keep cropping up. You don't know what to do or how to start. Plus, there's little time to set goals, much less achieve them.

Betsy McConnell is a clinical social worker who has worked with women for more than 20 years. "Many women today are stuck," she says. "They don't feel as if they have control over their lives," she adds. "They feel that the locus of control is external, not internal. I'm amazed at how little attention mothers give themselves. Women's lives are carried along by others. They have all the responsibility and not much power. The buck stops with them. They lack a vision of themselves as a separate person."

The answer may be to set an athletic goal. The word "goal" itself is a loaded word that can make you roll your eyes, feel uncomfortable right off the bat. Say it, and people may think "obsessive-compulsive", "daunting", "nitpicky", "phony", "oppressive", or even "here we go again."

Why the strong reaction? It's just a word, after all.

You (and they) may have set athletic goals in the past that fizzled. Perhaps the goals at the end of the day didn't hold your interests, fit with the logistics of your life, match your talents, deliver a congenial group of friends, whatever. Maybe you didn't really know how to set goals even though you thought you did. Things went wrong. Your schedule went out of control. You overdid it. You lost confidence in your goal – or even yourself – feeling that you weren't making progress or your goal wasn't realistic or you didn't have the support you needed, etc., etc., etc. Maybe the goal wasn't fun.

Or maybe you didn't have any goal – you just tried to "wing it", "go with the flow." That's what dental hygienist Milena Lopez did.

At 23, she started jogging for the first time. She said she had never been athletic but just wanted to be active. "I never had a weight issue but I didn't want to be a couch potato either," she said. "I wanted to get out there and enjoy the scenery." She began to jog for three minutes at a time. On the first day she jogged for a total of ten minutes with five minute walks between jogs. "Within a month of jogging three to four times a week I built up to 15 minutes in a row," she said.

Milena acknowledges that not having an athletic goal with structure just did not work over the long-term. "I didn't think I was making progress fast enough—and I didn't have anyone to run with, and then when the weather started getting cold, I didn't want to go out so I gave up at that point." That was about three years ago. "The problem with 'winging it' is that you can quit whenever you are tired instead of pushing yourself. I would just stop when I was tired. It was too easy to quit."

She also acknowledges that if she had a structured short-term goal with some kind of companionship or support and a way to recognize success in small steps of progress as in the *MOVE!* method, she would have continued. "Without structure and without anyone to jog with I had no more motivation," she said. She wishes she had known about *MOVE!* with its short-term goals and structured process to achievement.

Athletic Goal Defined

Of course, and to be clear at the outset, you don't have to run 50 miles a week to benefit from an athletic goal.

An athletic goal is *any* goal directed towards *any* physical challenge that

- *improves your current level of fitness* through a process of incremental training.
- *takes anywhere from six weeks* (the shortest term goal) to several years (long term goals).
- *has a "start" date to begin* training and *a "finish" date to complete it.*

For purposes of this book, an athletic goal must at least have a general definition. It could include walking one-half mile at the end of six weeks or completing a Hawaii Ironman. The goal simply has to represent something that you want to reach to improve your physical fitness and/or perform on a particular date. If you set a goal and it is an athletic goal, you are an athlete.

If your athletic goal is walking, you can improve by simply covering incrementally more distance and perhaps increasing your speed. A goal may involve other participants, like a race or tournament or swim for charity.....or not. Would competing in a croquet tournament be considered a goal? Yes – as long as it involves physical training and skill. A dance performance, a hike, a golf or tennis tournament can all be considered athletic goals if they fulfill the above criteria and involve training.

The word "athletic" reflects the fact that you are striving to improve. Don't be intimidated if you currently (erroneously) consider yourself a "non-athlete". Many women now in their 50s, 60s, and older grew up when people frowned on sports for girls and women – so some of you never had a chance to be athletic, even if you wanted to be. So, as a newly defined "athlete" or an experienced one, figure out your goal and define it based on your current fitness and interests. As soon as you choose your goal, you will feel more in control – and that, in itself, feels good, particularly when the rest of life makes you feel frazzled and often out of control.

Athletic Goals Under The Microscope

As I mentioned in the introduction, athletic goals are as likely as any category of goals to keep you balanced and focused but they also keep you strong and healthy. Several studies have shown that exercisers live longer than non-exercisers.

The microscope confirms the benefits. Exercise has been shown to affect us on a cellular and even molecular level. With exercise, the number of mitochondria in our cells increases even as we age. Mitochondria are the power centers of cells that provide the energy cells need to move, divide, secrete, and contract. Studies have shown that the more you exercise, and particularly the more intensely you exercise, the more mitochondria your cells have. The more mitochondria, the more endurance you have. You can run, cycle, or swim faster and longer.

Recent studies have also shown proof of the positive effects of exercise at the chromosomal level and specifically in telomeres – the ends of chromosomes – the structures which carry genes and which scientists believe are the biological clocks of cells impacting aging. Telomeres are the caps on the ends of chromosomes that protect against the unraveling of genes. They've been compared to caps on the ends of shoelaces. Every time cells divide, the telomeres get shorter. When the telomere get too short, the cells can no longer divide. When we age – when our muscles get weaker, hearing fades, or wrinkles appear – more cells reach the end of their telomeres and die. In one study, German scientists focused on 51-year-old male runners who ran more than 50 miles per week and found that their telomeres were almost the same length as those of 20-year-old runners on the German National Team and more than 40 percent longer than those of inactive men of the same age.[3]

---

3. Christian Werner, Tobias Fürster, Thomas Widmann, Janine Pöss, Cristiana Roggia, Milad Hanhoun, Jürgen Scharhag, Nicole Büchner, Tim Meyer, Wilfried Kindermann, Judith Haendeler, Michael Böhm, & Ulrich Laufs, "Physical Exercise Prevents Cellular Senescence in Circulating Leukocytes and in the Vessel Wall," Circulation 120 (2009), 2438-2447.

Another study of a group of 2,401 twins confirmed a positive association between telomere length and amount of exercise over a 10-year period.[4] People who exercised moderately – about 100 minutes a week of activity such as tennis, swimming, or running — had telomeres that on average looked like those of someone about five or six years younger than those who did the least — about 16 minutes a week. Those who did the most — about three hours a week of moderate to vigorous activity — had telomeres that appeared to be about nine years younger than those who did the least.

A test by physiologists of Olga Kotelko's muscle fibers (the nonagenarian track and field star referred to in the Introduction) found the unusual.[5] One would expect to see at least a few fibers with some mitochondrial defects in a person over 65. In 400 of Kotelko's fibers examined, however, not a single fiber showed evidence of mitochondrial defects.

The importance of written goals. My own research shows that 100% of the national- and world-class women runners set goals. Importantly, 96% of them wrote them down. In his book on Olympic athletes, The Pursuit of Sporting Excellence, author and Olympian David Hemery notes that 100% of Olympic athletes set specific goals.

The effectiveness of writing down goals was shown in a 1972 study involving Harvard Business School students. That year, 3% of the students said they had written down their goals and plans; 13% had no written goals; and 84% had no specific goals at all. Ten years later, in 1982, a follow up study found that the 13% who had goals but which were not written down earned, on average, twice as much as the 84% who had no goals. The 3% who wrote down their goals were earning 10 times the amount as the other 97% put

---

4. Lynn F. Cherkas, Janice L. Hunkin, Bernet S. Kato, J. Brent Richards, Jeffrey P. Gardner, Gabriela L. Surdulescu, Masayuki Kimura, Xiaobin Lu, Tim D. Spector, & Abraham Aviv, "The Association Between Physical Activity in Leisure Time and Leukocyte Telomere Length," Archives of Internal Medicine 168:2 (2008), 154-158.

5. Bruce Grierson, "The Incredible Flying Nonagenarian", The New York Times 25 November 2010.

together. [6] Whether you are uncomfortable or excited about goals, they help move you from a place of uncertainty to one of clarity. Setting goals and writing them down help provide structure. That in itself can be comforting and is an important step in figuring out just how to incorporate your goals into your hectic schedule.

Why Not Just Maintain A Fitness Routine?

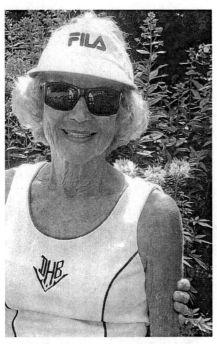

Diane Hoffman is always close to a tennis court.

The athletic goals are generally motivating and multidimensional than exercise routines, which can soon grow stale and boring. Not even champions feel like exercising without a purpose. New England Tennis Hall of Famer Diane Hoffman, who has won a world age group doubles championship and multiple national championships, says she still needs goals to motivate her every morning. Like most of us, she'd be more sedentary without them. "Without a goal of playing well for my teams I'd feel like going back to bed for the rest of the day and watching the tennis channel or Turner classic movies," she said.

With a goal, you're in control of identifying something that has meaning for you. Something as simple as practicing for a match can set off a chain of thinking that can lead to a new sense of purpose in life as a whole. So, an exercise routine may be a means to an end rather than the end itself. A goal makes the

---

6. Mark McCormack, What They Don't Teach You At The Harvard Business School (New York: Bantam Books, 1984).

exercise routine much more interesting. It (and you) has purpose. It will help you play your best, have more stamina, walk or swim further, etc.

Compared with fitness routines, athletic goals are more motivating and ultimately, rewarding. A goal requires you to build a training plan after which you're likely to reach peak fitness. You'll be stronger, faster, more flexible, more skilled, and leaner, most likely, than you'll be with an exercise routine alone. Say you decide your goal is to bike 10 miles in Vermont on a particular date. The moment you set it your thoughts jump to the weeks ahead. How will you start to build your miles? Will you lift weights? Will you improve your eating habits? Do you have the right equipment? Is your bike in good shape? As soon as you set your goal, you are motivated.

Because of the commitment and achievement involved in an athletic goal, it is more likely than mere routine to transform your outlook. Pursuing an athletic goal with the *MOVE!* method gives you a structure not just to transform your physical self but to realize other accomplishments as well. It helps you achieve balance in the rest of life.

Once Betsy McConnell understood the *MOVE!* method, she realized how different it is from working out in a gym. "This is a transformative process that changes your outlook on your whole life. Setting an athletic goal gives you a more positive vision than working out in a gym.

"Fitness is not about empowerment. It's about appearance. That's why I don't like the gym. It's about looking as good as you can. It's about pleasing other people. When you're an athlete, it's not about pleasing other people. It's about physical and psychological transformation."

As I said before, setting and achieving an athletic goal is such a concrete process that it provides an excellent learning experience for achieving other life goals. Want to restructure your career? Rethink an unhealthy relationship? Develop a new one? Start a new hobby? Once you learn the *MOVE!* method, you can use it in all areas of your life. After all, a goal is a goal is a goal. If you know how to apply principles of excellence and support and how to handle life's inevitable obstacles in the physical world, you can do the same in the rest of your life. Interestingly, after achieving their athletic goals, clients of mine have been inspired to change their careers, some have rethought unhealthy relationships and developed healthy ones, and some have started new hobbies. In reaching their athletic goals, these women have learned to set and manage goals in other parts of their life: how to apply principles of excellence, and how to handle life's inevitable hurdles and temporary setbacks, among other things.

The point? Achieving athletic goals is a powerful way to find balance, focus, control, discipline, connection, and freedom in your life as a whole. It's a way to gain confidence and a sense of calm that will help you relate to others. Pursuing athletic goals can help build the best friendships of your life. Sweat and trust go together.

Why For Women? Why Not Men?

The answer is that I am a woman, that I understand women's issues and that I have developed the *MOVE!* method over years of coaching women. It's true that I have used the system successfully

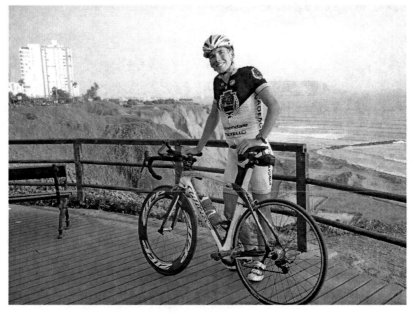

Joe Malloy before a triathlon in Lima, Peru

for male executives, college athletes, and coaches in my class "Elements of Competitive Performance" at Boston College. Joe Malloy, a former student and captain of Boston College's men's swim team is one athlete who has applied aspects of the *MOVE!* method to his training.

He asked why I was writing this book just for women. Now a professional triathlete and a member of the U.S. National Triathlon Team, Joe is travelling internationally to triathlons as he pursues his goal of making the 2012 Olympic Triathlon Team. He argued that *MOVE!* can work for men and their goals too. "This book and the *MOVE!* method speaks to the power of the human spirit," said Joe. "If you're determined to change yourself for the better-- it doesn't matter if you're young or old, male or female – this will resonate with you." This is absolutely true; but, as I mentioned above, the bulk of my experience, personal understanding, and enthusiasm comes from helping women attain their goals and – to paraphrase Eleanor Roosevelt – do the things they thought they could not do. The *MOVE!* method doesn't change who you are; it helps you to become the person you believe you can be.

Why Focus On Adults?

There is no structure available (or at least widely availed of) for adults after the high school or college community that encourages participation in teams or clubs. Because of this, it's easy for most adults to make excuses or rationalize their lack of exercise. We must create the structure for physical activity and figure out how to carve out time for it. (Yes. It is possible – even with your crazy schedule.)

For adults, much of the lack of simple exercise, much less athletic participation, is due not only to schedules but also to plain avoidance. Studies show that even mice tend to avoid exercise. Studies have also shown that goals build motivation to exercise even in the face of laziness or avoidance as well as difficulties, permanent or temporary disabilities and aging.[7] Therefore, as adults, goals can motivate us and challenge us to get out there, to exercise, and to rise to our physical potential.

It is important to understand that *MOVE!* takes this challenge to exercise beyond getting out on that treadmill. *MOVE!* asks you to set a goal in a certain physical activity – e.g. tennis, rowing, walking, hiking, sailing, biking, bowling – you name it – and then guides you to achieve that goal. After that, it's likely you'll be ready for your next goal, not to mention feel better about yourself. *MOVE!* is a method that actually gets you out there and, more importantly, keeps you out there which the metal, plastic, and rubber treadmill does not. *MOVE!* works to motivate you and keep you motivated.

So – When is the right time to take on an athletic goal?

---

7. Glyn Roberts, ed., Advances in Motivation in Sport & Exercise (Champaign, IL: Human Kinetics, 2001).

Any Time Can Be the Right Time

"I think the key for women is not to set any limits"
– Martina Navratilova

If you have little time, set small, manageable athletic goals.

In your 20s and 30s life can be unsettled. Athletic goals can keep you grounded.

In your 40s and 50s you may be taking care of others. Athletic goals encourage you to take time for yourself.

In your 60s, 70s, and beyond, you have more freedom. Pursue the athletic goals of your dreams.

You may be ill or have experienced tough times. Athletic goals can bring you unexpected happiness.

So, you know you want to take on an athletic goal. You're ready psychologically. Is there an optimal time or stage in life to actually start? No, there isn't. Today may be a great day to start. *Any time, any decade,* can be the right time. It can be right when things in your life are going well – or when they aren't. What if you have very little time? *Don't abandon your dream of your goal because of a busy schedule.* Just set smaller, more manageable goals that put you on the road to the larger one.

Our lives are all busy, complex, unique. However, certain challenges and patterns are more typical of some ages than others.

20s, 30s – Athletic Goals Provide An Anchor And Network

During these decades you're close to your peak physiological potential, so it's a great time to seize the moment. In our twenties and thirties, however, many of us are also trying to either define ourselves or establish ourselves. Relationships and careers may be unsettled at this point. Experts are now recognizing the twenties as one of life's most stressful decades for just those reasons. Thus, for those in their twenties and thirties, an athletic goal can serve as an anchor in a time of uncertainty and stress and as a vehicle for expanding your network of friends and associates.

It did for Barbara Bellesi, who – like many women in their twenties – was "at sea" in her career. She had left her job of several years teaching eighth grade English and was working several part-time jobs as a writer. "I was in the middle of a career change and was looking for something that had specific goals that I could mark off. Things were still uncertain in my life…. I didn't know where my career was going, and I wanted an accomplishment that I could be sure of and something that I could always have with me regardless of where I went. Because I am not a marathon runner or a runner to begin with, I wanted something that was specific for my ability." She chose a three-day, 60 mile walk for breast cancer as her goal.

Barbara was looking for an anchor in her life and achieving

this walk meant control, achievement, and confidence. "Achieving this goal reinforced my confidence in working towards any goal. I felt strong and better able to go after jobs and relationships." Mallory Champa, an All-American and former Division 1 runner now in her twenties, agrees that the twenties can be a time of uncertainty. "In the first years after college, you are not yet settled and a lot can feel unsettled in terms of your career, where you're living, and personal life. It's up to you to figure out a structure. *MOVE!* can help you discover and implement your priorities."

An athletic goal can also help you establish yourself by expanding your network of friends or professional associates. Networks are important if you've just moved to a new city, started a new career, or decided to work towards a promotion.

Melissa Deland set a new athletic goal in her late twenties for multiple reasons. It would be fun and she always had an "athletic drive". She also thought her goal would help her build a professional network.

At 25, while working in residential real estate sales, she took up golf. "I had a flexible schedule and golf was something I could do on my own," she said. "I also needed an outlet for my athletic drive and I wanted something I could fit into my schedule." She

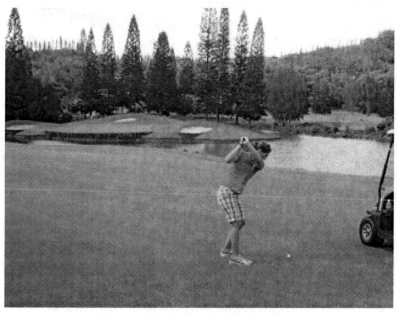

Melissa Deland going for the green.

was also single and wanting to make business connections to help her career. Her father had been a good golfer. "I was intrigued by playing an individual sport," she added.

"In my first sales job I had some hours between appointments so I would drive around and find public golf courses and go to driving ranges. If I had 2 hours, I would play 9 holes," she said. "It helped me network for my business career. I had never used athletics to further my career, and I made a handful of important connections on the golf course. Golf gave me an arena for connecting with others in the business."

40s, 50s – Athletic Goals For "Me Time", Sanity, A Sense of Direction

In her forties and fifties, who doesn't feel overwhelmed from time to time with responsibilities? We're managing households, jobs, relationships, volunteer efforts – you name it. Many of us in these decades feel the pressures of "care", sandwiched between two major care responsibilities such as children and aging parents or whomever. "I need some time for myself!", "I need to come up for air", or "I need to slow things down and take a breath" are comments of women commonly heard that reflect the general feelings of these decades.

Remember how airlines tell all adult passengers with children to put an oxygen mask on themselves first and then on their children? An athletic goal – even a small goal, one that might require an hour three times a week – just might be your oxygen mask. The training – even if it's walking – will be good for your mental and physical health and, most likely, make you more productive and effective in your responsibilities.

Connie Kowalski's and Betsy Shields' experiences as mothers are different, but equally compelling examples of women whose athletic goals reinforced perspective and saved them at a time when they were both in the vortex of responsibilities and caring for others.

At 45, Connie found herself overwhelmed, balancing a

full-time job as a legal secretary with marriage and parenting three children, ages 12, 14, and 15. "Life was crazy", she said. "I depended on other parents to help drive my kids to soccer practice. Between my husband, who works as a contractor (so his hours are erratic – sometimes he works late, and sometimes early), we had little free time. We tried to make up for it on week-ends which we'd then devote entirely to the kids."

Connie found herself, at 45, about 25 pounds overweight and concerned when she felt breathless after climbing a flight of stairs. "I knew I had to get my body into shape just for health reasons," she said.

Picking an athletic goal was challenging for two reasons. First, Connie had never been involved in sports. "I was the member of Girl Scouts who loved canoeing and hiking, but I was never coordinated and I steered away from competitive sports at all costs." Second, she had little time, with managing a household and working from 9 to 5 five days a week.

She hired a trainer at a gym and set a six-week goal of walking three miles at a time. On three of five work days she walked (and rested) for 30 minutes during her lunch hour. She walked as well on Saturdays and Sundays.

"I got a lot 'done' during my walks – a lot of productive, creative thinking about work and my family. Sometimes I missed meeting a friend for lunch, but often I'd convince that person to walk with me. Just the process of training to walk three miles at a time made me feel in control of my time and health. Maybe I will do a charity walk sometime."

Betsy is a mother of four girls. Between 29 and 37, Shields was either nursing babies or pregnant. She had given up her paid career to care for her daughters, although she continued to volunteer for two land trusts. Athletic all her life and a swimmer in college, she stayed fit during those years by walking, biking, running, and swimming, but she was not focused on any goals – not until her youngest was two.

"When my youngest was two, I finally had enough sleep and enough time to take on a mini-triathlon. It was a low commitment, low pressure, very neighborly event."

She found that pursuing an athletic goal gave her time for herself as well as a sense of direction. "Negotiating with kids all day long and absorbing all of their tantrums and stress and testing encourages you to find some release – you need to leave them and do something for yourself so you can get rid of all that stress that you're holding.

"It also gave me something to work towards. It's useful to have something to work for even it's small and low pressure. Often you say you're going to learn how to ride a road bike and you don't....particularly if it's a little uncomfortable. A goal got me more focused on going for a real workout."

How did she manage mini-triathlon training with four daughters between 2 and 10? She'd be up at 5 AM when they were sleeping or, if she got out later, grandparents or a babysitter would watch the girls. Training for the mini-triathlon gave her "mental space" and sanity, she said. "It allowed me to recharge and to feel as if I was moving forward at the same time."

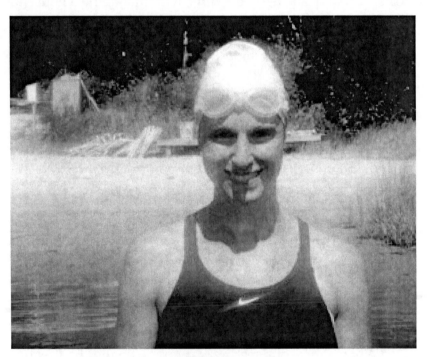

Betsy Shields after a swim.

60s, 70s, and Beyond – Athletic Goals Realize A Lifetime Dream

You've worked for years. Maybe you've raised a family. Finally, you have more freedom. You may even have saved up some money to travel. In your sixties, seventies, and beyond, you may want to set a dream goal. Again, it can be as simple as walking or hiking. You may train to walk a mile by the end of the month.

Having been widowed at 51, Carrie Parsi worked as a registered nurse to raise three children. She had always set athletic goals. Turning 60 and 70 were occasions to take on two of the most challenging athletic goals of her life. "It was a way of rewarding myself for reaching these ages. I felt grateful that I was still strong and I wanted to celebrate the freedom I had at these stages in life. When you have children, you can't just drop them and take off. There's less freedom to train and travel. Reaching the higher ages frees you up from a lot of responsibility – from family…so there's a sense of independence when it comes to older ages. It's not so easy to pull up when you're 30 or 40 even for a three day trip. Part of the satisfaction is that you've waited – your family or jobs are pretty much completed. Being older allows you to challenge yourself more without worrying about what happens."

At 60, she ran the Inca Trail in Peru. "It was a privilege to be on that trail," she said. "There was something historical about the whole setting. Coming into Machu Pichu at the end of the day was awesome."

At 70, she took advantage of her fitness to achieve her longtime dream of climbing Mt. Kilimanjaro – the most challenging goal of her life. Other than Parsi, the youngest person on the trip was 56. "It was the toughest thing I've ever done," said Parsi. "But it was just amazing. We got up to the summit in time for the sunrise over Kilimanjaro."

Any Decade – Athletic Goals When Life is Not Going So Well

You don't usually consider an athletic goal when you're not feeling your best – but sometimes it can be the best thing to do. If you're feeling bored, "down", or anxious, an athletic goal can energize and calm you at the same time – and give you a feeling of a "jump start" on life. Even if you have a temporary or chronic physical disability, you might find that an athletic goal revives you in ways you never imagined. Taking the first step may be the hardest thing to do because it may feel counterintuitive when you're not feeling strong. But suspend belief and try. Take a step and go for it.

Sue Gustafson and Karin Miller are two women who took on athletic goals when they were fighting lows. In her mid-forties, Sue found herself in a "nasty, deep depression" following a relationship that had not worked out. She eventually took up running. At 35, Karin was diagnosed with rheumatoid arthritis. Though she moves with unusual grace, both hands are slightly gnarled. She started martial arts. Through their pursuits, both Sue and Karin transformed their lives.

"I was literally crippled by the depression," said Sue. "I was having problems with my job and life. At one point I was literally curled up under my desk at work. I felt I would never have a chance at love again. I felt completely incompetent and worthless."

Despite these feelings and the fact that she had never been athletic – "I had always been the intellectual and artistic one" – she managed to start running a few days a week, building up to three miles at a time. "Everybody's depression is different. Mine had light spots mixed in with the black, and there were enough light spots that I could drag myself out on the road once a day." Friends helped. A group of co-workers started running together. That became a habit and then she realized she could do more distance than she thought. Before she knew it, she started doing longer runs.

"Starting a goal as the crisis eased physically managed

the residual depression. The training kicked in the endorphins. The goal helped me believe in myself. I had more strength than I thought and I realized that I could gain strength that only special people had. The training certainly didn't cure the depression but it gave me a sense of accomplishment and made me feel capable of something big at a time when I needed it most. As I came out of the depression, it gave me something to hold on to and it helped establish some competence, control, and worth. I couldn't deny that I had accomplished something I tried to do.

"I would highly recommend some kind of physical goal to anyone who's feeling that they are emerging from their depression. An athletic goal is like a brail trail. It's like knots in a rope you can hold on to. It helps you get something into perspective. It's something positive you can achieve each day. It gives you a sense of control. Any sense of control is huge."

All of her life, Karin Miller had taken physical activity for granted. She had always been a strong skier, swimmer, tennis player, and runner. Moving painlessly was something she simply did, without thought or deliberation. Suddenly, in her early thirties, specific joints began not to just ache, but to cause pain that rendered them unusable. Over the years, the pain worsened. Movement became more and more of a challenge. "When you find yourself thinking long and hard about what it will take to actually move a couple of body parts or joints you find yourself facing a challenge that can be devastating, overwhelming, and humiliating," she said. "I was almost never out of a flare-up. My spleen used to be palpable, it was so enlarged."

"When you've been physical much of your life and your body's done whatever it's been asked to do, and you do things reasonably well, you can't quite imagine what it would be like not be able to do much of anything physical without significant discomfort and pain. Most of my life, I never thought about moving. I just moved." Regular exercise, as she had known it, and over the counter medications anyone would take for inflammation did not alleviate the pain.

"It's never easy when your body lets you down," Karin continued. "In my case, I was embarrassed. I had always been a 'can do' kind of person. It got to the point where I had to think long and hard about whether even the most basic of activities was a remote possibility."

Then, she decided to try what she calls a "mind-body connection experiment"; she hoped that if she exercised her mind and body in a disciplined, focused way, her symptoms might improve. At 44, she tried Moo Do, a Korean martial art. "It was something that I had never done before – something that could not happen without deliberate thought and focus."

At first she felt completely ill at ease, "in a strange environment with people in strange outfits." But thinking the training might help her pain, she persisted – to the point where for five years she trained six times a week, usually for several hours at a time.

Between ages 45 and 52 she had only one flare-up. "I can lead a full, active, rich pain-free life," she asserts. Her doctors are stunned.

"Looking back, what I was searching for was what is now so commonly referred to as being in touch with the 'mind-body' connection," she said.

"Now, she said, "being physical in a very deliberate and thoughtful way has become a way of life. Keeping my mind and my thoughts positive and focused is key. The additions of yoga, Pilates, cycling and even a mindful walk outdoors are part of daily routines that not only keep an ailment or possible disability at bay but also become significant steps toward helping me move in the direction of my next physical goal – healthy aging."

The *MOVE!* Method

*"The future belongs to those who believe
in the beauty of their dreams."*
– Eleanor Roosevelt

*MOVE! is a simple, versatile goal achievement method that helps
you identify realistic athletic goals given everything else in your
life.*

*There are five practical steps to achieving your goal with
MOVE!: (1) prepare for goals (2) set realistic goals (3) manage
the process (4) assess the outcome and (5) set the next goal.*

*Five things to keep in mind, the "underlying guidelines", are:
(1) see the big picture (2) enter the "beginner's mind" (3) have
support (4) focus your practice and (5) remember that mastery
takes time.*

*MOVE! goes beyond athletics. You can use MOVE! for personal
and professional goals as well.*

The main reason I created the *MOVE!* method was that I was looking for a system of achieving goals for myself and for the athletes I was coaching and couldn't find anything that seemed to work. Since it's a method that has subsequently worked for me and for others, I'm confident it will be helpful to you. Setting goals is great, but achieving them is another matter. It can be hard to figure out what they might or should be – particularly when we're comfortable with the status quo. The mere idea of goal setting is challenging but it does tempt us to experiment, reach, change, and ask "What if?".

Where do we learn about goal setting, generally? Maybe at work (trying to make sales quotas), in a psychology or business course, on a sports team? Few people – including student athletes and college sports captains – know how to set goals that actually work. The coaches do that for them. Ask them to set a goal on their own, and they're taken aback. "We've never worked one-on-one with the coaches on in-depth goals," said one college track team captain. "In the beginning of the season everyone wrote down a seasonal goal and I thought it should be something that my coach would want to hear. I became frustrated because I didn't know how to translate my goals into actions and get results. I set them without really looking at myself and my situation."

"When you're part of a team, your goals blend together with others and they're not your unique goal," says Acacia Walker, a Boston College lacrosse coach and also a member of the World Cup Lacrosse Team for the past 10 years. "When you get outside of that team, you wonder what the next goal is. It may be the first time you define your own personal goal that fits into your life. Having a structure like *MOVE!* allows you to think about your own goals and build a plan to achieve them."

Explaining The Method

MOVE! is a method of goal setting and achievement that can help you identify new, meaningful athletic and other life goals, translate them into action, and reach them. It puts you in the

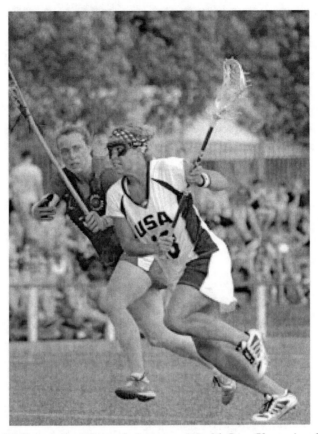

Acacia Walker at the Women's Lacrosse World Cup Championships.
PHOTOGRAPH BY JOSEPH WALKER.

driver's seat, helps you enjoy the process, avoid distraction, and stay on track. Once you are in control of your direction, you feel *motivated*. With training books, calendars and successive, short-term goals that build to a longer term goal, *MOVE! organizes* you. It encourages you to picture your ideal future. *Visualize*, then realize. With forms focused on overcoming obstacles and evaluating goal achievement, *MOVE!* helps you *excel*. Most importantly, *MOVE!* condenses time to achievement and incorporates setbacks and even failure as part of learning and ultimate success.

The MOVE! method is a versatile five step process for achieving your athletic goals.

MOVE!'s (and your) success is based on the theory that achieving goals is a matter not just of setting goals and winging it – more often than not, a recipe for failure – but instead

- making sure you are prepared for the goal before you set it,
- setting specific short- and long-term goals,
- managing the process,
- once you've achieved your goal, assessing the overall process, and
- setting the next goal.

Each of the five practical steps of preparing, setting, managing, assessing, and setting the next goal is discussed in detail later in the book but here is a brief overview of each.

The Five Practical Steps of *MOVE!*

1: Prepare for Goals

- Consider everything going on in your life on a monthly as well as weekly basis, and
- consider the athletic options that make the most sense (and are most fun) for you.

2: Set Goals

- Develop a vision of how you see yourself when you achieve your goal,
- identify and confront doubts and fears, and
- set successive short-term goals of six to ten weeks and, if you want, annual goals.

3: Manage the Process

- Keep a training log by writing training records in a journal and using a three-month training calendar for perspective,

• keep a weekly appointment with yourself,
•enjoy weekly support (talking/e-mailing/Skyping/training) with a buddy which makes the process more fun and fulfilling,
• consult a coach or experienced athlete for advice, and
• face inevitable setbacks, new and old doubts and fears head-on to help you "reset" or modify your goal in some way, to give you the necessary flexibility to stay on course to achieve the goal.

4: Assess your Achievement

• Review your achievements – or temporary non-achievements – whether they're of interim short-term goals, annual goals, or after a major event (which may be neither a short-term or annual goal). We all too often forget *the process* that leads to achievement. Assessing the process can tell you a lot about what went right and what went wrong, and what you'd like to improve in the future toward your current or next goal.

5: Set the Next Goal

• Congrats – you've achieved your overall goal. Now is the time to keep your momentum going by building on the same goal (run a 10K now that you've run a 5K) or change your sport or activity now that you've run a 5K successfully. Put away the bike for a while and learn to row or hike the Presidentials. If you have trouble shifting sports, *MOVE!* suggests straightforward steps to help you let go of the old and attempt something new, something even equally rewarding and productive. It's hard, sometimes, to say you're done with a sport or activity. Letting go and trying something new is often energizing. In addition to your athletic goals, you may be just as energized by taking on a wholly new venture such as writing that book you've wanted to for so long. As far as activities (athletic and non-athletic) go, the sky's the limit.

Underlying Guidelines

So we've discussed the five practical steps to achieving your goals. The steps are supported by five underlying guidelines and they're discussed in depth in the next chapter. They make goal achievement much easier.

The underlying guidelines are:
• see the big picture,
• enter the "beginner's mind",
• have support,
• focus your practice, and
• remember that mastery takes time.

MOVE! Is A Fluid Method

What do I mean when I say *MOVE!* is a fluid method? Depending on your background, you may hire a coach from the start or perhaps on just an occasional basis. When you want to work with a "buddy" is up to you.

Paradoxically, the method works precisely because it is fluid. It recognizes that preparing, managing, reviewing, and modifying goals are as vital to their achievement as setting them. <u>All five practical steps are important!</u> They may be modified and shaped to fit your life and your goals, but the five steps themselves are important. Skipping one may affect your ability to achieve your ultimate goal. So, work within the system as you wish, but don't ignore the constituent parts.

The Forms

Importantly, the five practical steps to achieving your goals with the *MOVE!* method are reinforced by completing simple forms, critical to the process and helpful for guidance and record keeping. Why are they important? I know. Forms are a bore. Most people don't like filling out forms. Don't worry. As I've said, it's a flexible process. But the forms are easy to complete and do provide a concrete method to demonstrate what you have accomplished and what you need to accomplish. You can't track what you can't measure. Finally, they help ensure your commitment to your goal. The forms are an intrinsic part of the overall *MOVE!* method. Remember the Harvard MBA study where the 3% who wrote down their goals earned more than the other 97% altogether?

MOVE! – Beyond Athletic Goals

Understanding the versatility of *MOVE!* will help you see how you can apply it to other aspects of your life, not just athletic goals. As mentioned, while people have used the method for their athletic goals, some have subsequently used it for their career and their personal goals. And frankly, there are times in our lives when we just are not able to set athletic goals – times when certain circumstances do prevent us temporarily from taking them on. (I would emphasize temporarily.) The power of the *MOVE!* method, however, is that it works for all of life's goals. Jenny is an example of a woman who used the method for a non-athletic goal, and her story is worth telling as it may help you read the following chapters on athletic goals with a broader perspective.

Jenny is a friend – one of those new/old or old/new friends, by which I mean that I met her just two years ago, and we were sure we had met before though we both also knew we hadn't. We felt totally "in sync" (maybe it was the faded red polo shirt and the old style jeans). She represents that group of women who has benefited and will benefit from this book in ways beyond athletics. Jenny was a high-level athlete in college (a nationally ranked squash player all four years), active since college in a number of sports (snow boarding, golf, etc.) since college, and she ran fairly regularly. She held a high-powered job in London for many years while being married and raising two daughters.

Along with significant successes, however, she experienced

one of the greatest tragedies a mother can. Months after returning to the US from London, her older daughter, Casey, 13, was diagnosed with a brain tumor. Casey died days after her fourteenth birthday. Jenny obviously continues to grieve. We spoke a while ago and she felt she hadn't accomplished much since Casey died. "I feel as if I am one of those cartoon characters who are above the ravine trying to get back to land – and their feet and legs are moving frantically and they could fall in at any moment but haven't yet. Despite the frantic motion, the character isn't moving forward." The one project she did take on was to renovate their newly purchased house. It required moving out, renting another place, and moving back in. (And she thought she hadn't accomplished anything!) She had thought of the renovation and moves as a pain-in-the-rear interruption in her life.

It was actually in a conversation with Jenny that I first realized – months after having started writing this book – the multifaceted essence of its message, i.e., *MOVE!*'s application beyond athletic goals.

I had asked if taking on an athletic goal would in any way help her recover? I knew she hadn't even been exercising regularly with all of the turmoil in her life.

"Take on an athletic goal?" she said to me incredulously, sitting amidst dozens of unopened boxes in her new kitchen. "I can't imagine taking on one now. I am mired in this move – and I'm still an emotional wreck.

"You're right," I said. "It's not the right time for that now. An athletic goal can wait until your move is finished."

Then I thought about her move and the *MOVE!* method. Why not use it for her move? "You've read the draft of my book," I said. "What about reorienting your thinking and considering your move not as an interruption to be endured but as an achievement? A move is just as much of a goal as a physical one is." She could apply any or all of the steps of the *MOVE!* goal setting method to the rest of her move. She could set successive short-term goals, write a vision statement, find a buddy, overcome the obstacles, and celebrate completing the move. Taking at least some of the steps would help her strategize and see the move as a project to be mastered. She might then regard the drudgery as discipline which would make an accomplishment out of an obligation. In my process, there's a Post-Goal Analysis that helps you reflect back on how you achieved your goal and it helps you validate the process and give yourself credit for it.

Of course I liked the idea, and Jenny agreed that the method could energize her and help her achieve the move faster than if she saw it as an annoying distraction. She'd feel more in control. The process might even be fun.

Jenny applied the method successfully to her move, getting it done more quickly than she planned and enjoying it more. With my encouragement, she started running again more regularly. She is now about to begin that athletic goal we talked about. Her motivation has begun to return.

Once a 12 handicap in golf, but not having played much since kids arrived 16 years ago, Jenny wants to get back to her previous level and see if she can lower her handicap to single digits. A good round requires muscle tone, stamina, a positive attitude, and hours and hours of practice. So Jenny is about to begin an active workout schedule in addition to actual practice.

"*MOVE!* has already made an impact on my life – mentally, emotionally and physically. Its method of realistic goal setting and achievement has given me a real gift in making the daunting do-able, the improbable possible and achievable," she said. "In addition to golf, I may even think seriously about writing a book on a topic I've been pondering for some time. If I do, I'll definitely use the *MOVE!* method to get it done."

So you can see that *MOVE!* can apply to all sorts of goals, athletic, non-athletic, short-term, long-term, etc., and energize you in the process. More on that but let's return for now to the underlying guidelines of *MOVE!*. You'll have a better sense of why it works.

Underlying Guidelines

"An overnight success usually takes about ten years."
- Anonymous

Seeing the big picture helps you consider all your life commitments before setting an athletic goal.

Entering the "beginner's mind" encourages you to experiment and enter your "no comfort" zone.

Finding support reminds you that you need a cheering section.

Focusing your practice means practice should be specific, and targeted to your weaknesses as well as strengths.

Remembering that "mastery takes time" teaches you that excellence requires patience – as much as 10 years (10,000 hours).

This chapter discusses the underlying guidelines mentioned in the previous chapter, guidelines for what you must keep in mind as you pursue your athletic goals.

As with most successful endeavors in life, it pays to think things out rather than act impulsively or just jump in the middle with no plan. Say you want to build a house. First, you need an overall plan. You don't want the plumber to show up before you build the foundation. You want to build a foundation that's the right size. With the athletic goals you've set for yourself, the process is just the same. Guidelines are an important part of that foundation of goal achievement, as they help you with the right expectations, direction, and pace. With *MOVE!* they're essential, and they explain why it consistently helps people succeed. As mentioned previously, to achieve your goal, whatever it is, you need to train in a coherent manner with both big and, importantly, smaller goals along the way which add up to the big one. With such a plan, you'll have more patience with yourself and feel success as you achieve your interim and final goals. And guess what? You'll probably reach them faster.

The Five Underlying Guidelines

Again, the five essential guidelines or things to keep in mind to achieve your goals are:

- See the big picture
- Enter the "beginner's mind"
- Find support
- Focus your practice, and
- Remember: Mastery takes time.

1: See The Big Picture
Before you pick a goal, consider everything in your life – your health, work, family, relationships, community, household, etc. How many commitments do you currently have and is there time for another one? In my study of master women runners (women runners over 40), the greatest obstacle to their success – a

greater obstacle than injuries or the effects of menopause – was too many commitments. Here's a suggestion: if you already have more than three major priorities or commitments in life, assess whether it really is a good time to set a physical goal.

My rule of thumb is that, for most women, four goals or commitments that include your athletic goal is the maximum that you can manage without going crazy. This does not contradict my previous statement about crazy schedules not being an impediment. Schedules *always* can be altered to fit an athletic goal. A priority or commitment can't. So if you have five or more commitments including the athletic goal you probably need to wait or to scale back on your athletic goal. None of these statements should make you think – or give you a reason – not to undertake an athletic goal. Exercise will help you take on your other commitments positively and with greater energy. Just realistically assess them and plan accordingly. Here is an example of a woman with many commitments who has scaled back temporarily on her overall athletic goal.

In many respects, Annmarie O'Brien is a woman with responsibilities typical of those of others in their mid-forties. A national masters track and field silver medalist in her age group, she hasn't thought about an ambitious goal in a national championship for years – and for good reason. "Running for me has been about not getting too stressed." She is married with two active children whom she drives to lacrosse, ballet, and numerous other activities. She works full-time as a legal secretary. She and her siblings work together to take care of her octogenarian parents who live 15 minutes away. Both her parents have Alzheimer's disease and still live in their own house.

"I set up the appointments and my sister takes them….For example, both of my parents have to have cataract surgery, both eyes each…. My brother cooks for them on Sundays," she said. "Tomorrow I am meeting with a woman whom I hired to go in three days a week….I am also redoing my parents' bathroom."

Like Annmarie, many of us have to juggle several balls. Like many of us, Annmarie has had to reduce the number of events and intensity of athletic goals she's striving for in order to maintain life balance. She sees the big picture and sees that, for now, the appropriate course is to pursue less competitive goals.

"It's not easy to put the training aside when you have a lot on your plate….but it's so much better mentally," she said.

When you find yourself at a point when you *are* able to take on a new athletic goal, saying "no" to some other commitments is critical to success. And that's not easy. It's particularly hard when you're used to accommodating and helping others – friends, family, and colleagues. And, frankly, many women have a tough time saying "no" to others and putting themselves first.

When deciding on your athletic goal, you should also ask yourself how much time, money, and effort you want to invest as part of the big picture. You may just want to learn tennis well enough to play doubles at a beginner level. You may want to walk a mile….or you may have found a sport you want to excel in. Finally, ask yourself what does achieving a new goal mean to you? What is it that you really want to accomplish overall?

2: Enter the "Beginner's Mind"

Once you have decided on your athletic goal, remembering the virtues of what Zen Buddhism calls the "beginner's mind" helps you start your goal – particularly if you're used to being competent and in control in your life. This is important. You may feel nervous about being a novice again – so give yourself credit for entering the "beginner's mind" and experimenting. How do you do that?

> • Let go being an expert – of knowing,
> • Remind yourself that you learn by mistakes, by falling down,
> • Let go of "shoulds" or "once I could haves",
> • Focus on performing the activity and forget outside observers, including yourself (this is no place for self-con sciousness), and
> • Focus on questions, not answers.

My own experience fits here. Sidelined from running by an injury in my late forties, I felt restless. I thought about an athletic goal that would still allow me to recover appropriately from my injury. My husband is an avid sailor, my kids enjoy sailing, I wasn't a sailor, but we had just bought a sailboat. The truth was

I had always hated sailing. I grew pale at the slightest rocking. I have a hard time understanding mechanical parts. Those are "meat and potatoes" in sailing. It takes me a while to figure out how to put the DVD into the DVD player. Concerned about being a "boater's widow", however, (other women had warned me about this), I decided to enter the "beginner's mind" and earn a certification to sail a small boat. Just because I didn't feel comfortable on a boat didn't mean I couldn't master one.

So I flew to Annapolis, Maryland for a week-long sailing course at J World. That's an intensive, Outward Bound-style sailing school known for its rigor and aimed at rewarding its graduates with a keel boat certification to sail any boat up to 27 feet. Cool – I thought – I'll be walking my talk as a coach. I was proud of my status as a beginner in a sport that stressed my weaknesses and felt as if I'd already accomplished my goal when I stepped on the plane.

I was quickly in my no-comfort zone. Confined in a 26-foot boat from 9:30 to 4:30, I couldn't move as much as I liked. I had to ask more times than others which line the halyard was. In man overboard drills I had to repeat to myself out loud – ignoring what others might have thought. In fact, they didn't mind at all.... Some of them began doing the same thing.

In the end, I earned my certification and felt immensely rewarded. First, I had thought I would always get seasick on a boat, and I didn't. Second, I actually enjoyed sailing, which meant more fun time with my family on weekend excursions. Third, I wasn't as bad as I thought with instructions and mechanical parts like boom vangs and cunninghams. The point? The thought of being a beginner did not keep me from going to sailing school. Entering the "beginner's mind" was essential and not a turn off.

Once you've decided to become a beginner again, don't be afraid of stumbling, even failing. In my sailing course, I told myself I could make mistakes because I knew I'd learn more from making than avoiding them. As an example, on the first day I volunteered to raise the sail. I pulled on a line (rope) that did nothing of the kind, and then pulled on another line that also did nothing. So I sat down, took a breath, and surveyed the lines slowly. I didn't feel too smart. I wondered if the instructor was watching. "But that's ok," I told myself. "You're a good person and, yes, you are a beginner. You can make mistakes." With patience, I did find the halyard, the line used to hoist the sail, even if it took me longer than others. After that, I never forgot where it was.

3: Find Support

No matter what we do in life, who doesn't need social support? According to University of Chicago research psychologist John Cacioppo, such support is essential for health alone. In his 2008 landmark book, Loneliness, Cacioppo compiled 30 years of research that showed that lack of social support – loneliness – can be harmful to well-being, including physical health. Those who are lonely, for example, are likely to have higher blood pressure and weaker immune systems than those with social supports.

From the perspective of achieving your athletic goal, support from others is a critical motivator for success. Friendships, according to authors Carole Holahan and Robert Sears (The Gifted Group in Later Maturity, 1995), motivated over a thousand successful professionals (men and women most of whom were in their sixties and seventies) more than money or status. In Good to Great (2001), a study of companies which became stand-outs in their fields, business consultant Jim Collins echoed the importance of friendships as critical motivators: "The people we interviewed," he wrote, "….clearly loved what they did largely because they loved who they did it with."

Everyone needs support even when life is smooth. Setbacks abound. Injuries, doubts, disappointments, and other distractions invariably rear their ugly heads. Who doesn't lose faith, sometimes, or feel angry and just want to quit? Support in some form is essential to achievement. Whether you're a beginner or Olympian, real support can be tricky to find. Sometimes people you think should support you – teammates, your family, your friends – don't. In fact, they may compete with you or unconsciously undermine you. They might not think your time is well spent on your sport. They may resent your time away from them. To succeed, we need at least one person who has our interests at heart.

What is support anyway? It depends. It can be emotional empathy (a sounding board), technical (advice from a coach), or logistical (a ride to the pool, babysitting).

It turns out that emotional support is usually more important than technical support in achieving your athletic goal. In my doctoral study of 103 masters women runners, 70% attributed their success to verbal support from coaches, whereas 82% attributed success to verbal support from family and friends.[8] A study of 170 NCAA Division I college athletes on technical and emotional support delivered similar results.[9] The athletes relied on support from friends more than twice as often as they did support from coaches.

Recognizing support can be challenging. You may find it in another athlete, but you may not. You may find it in a neighbor, a sibling, a non-athlete, friend, a former teacher – or even a pet.

So – how do you find support? Look for a feeling of interest, sincerity, and goodwill. Former Olympian Carol Skricki discussed the challenge of finding support. Carol started rowing at age 31 and made the 2000 Olympic team at age 38. She gives some valuable advice:

"Pay attention to all the support around. The power of one person's support can be huge. You have to be able to recognize what you should be grabbing onto as it goes by and following the positive people and not following the draining, negative stuff."

Carol stresses the importance of saying "no" to people who drag you down, and "yes" to those who lift you up. "You have to say 'no' to some things," she said. "You have to have a gut feeling about what to say 'yes' to. It's not worth calling up people who are subtly going to undermine you or your confidence, who are going to make you feel down when you hang up the phone. It's hard when you want them to be your friends."

Carol also pointed out the advantage of finding emotional support outside of your sport. "You may also find emotional support outside the physical arena," she said. " It's good to have friends who are not part of the rowing world. Friends who are

---

8. Catharine Utzschneider, Women Runners Who Became National Caliber After Age 40 (Ann Arbor: ProQuest Information and Learning, 2002).

9. Lawrence B. Rosenfeld, Jack M. Richman, & Charles J. Hardy, "Examining social support networks among athletes: Description and relationship to stress," The Sport Psychologist 3 (1989), 23-33.

recreational rowers or not rowers at all can be the best supporters. They see your situation objectively."

It's important to get support from family or those you live with and sometimes it takes longer than you think to get it. Don't expect to get it right away. Family members will have to adjust, and they may doubt that you'll really stick with your goal if they haven't seen you committed before and even tell you so. Best thing to do: tell them you need them to help you. Chances are they'll respond positively.

When you hear of women achieving their athletic dreams, chances are they've had a great deal of support from home. Carolyn Smith-Hanna is a masters runner who has achieved world records in two age groups, women 50 to 54 and women 55 to 59. A physical education teacher, wife, and mother of two, she described the critical importance of support from home: "Does my husband support me? My husband was a cross-country champion in high school in 1968. He has taken over dinner, done more than his share of housework. He has gone out of his way to allow me to train. He has to fend for himself for two nights a week. I don't know how I could do this without him. If he resented my doing that, it would have made this very difficult."

The truth is, we don't always have a spouse or partner or roommate who agrees to pick up a portion of household responsibilities, but Carolyn's point is important. Someone else was encouraging her to achieve her athletic goal without direct input into the actual goal. Her husband's support facilitated and therefore greatly enhanced Carolyn's chances of success.

4: Focus Your Practice

There's nothing wrong with general practice. With general practice, though, we tend not to focus on our weaknesses. They're not as much fun, but if you want to improve in a sport, you have to focus on your strengths <u>and</u> your weaknesses. You have to engage in "deliberate practice", a concept developed by Dr. K. Anders Ericsson, Professor at Florida State University and one of the world's leading theoretical and experimental researchers on expertise.[10]

Deliberate practice is aimed at reaching goals just beyond your present level of competence. In deliberate practice you focus on your weaknesses and specific needs, you repeat your exercises many times but continually adjust them in accordance with feedback from a coach or teacher. Throughout all this you must concentrate a great deal and not get frustrated.

Here's an example of the difference between practice and deliberate practice. A golfer might practice putting by randomly placing three or four balls on the putting green at a time and working on hitting them into the hole for maybe 15 minutes. By contrast, Lisa, is an experienced golfer with a low handicap, who focuses her practice – or practices deliberately.

"Putting," she said, "has always been difficult for me. I used to dread getting to the green in a tournament, because then I would have to putt. Deliberate practice drills sharpen my game without the mental and physical fatigue that comes with playing a round of golf..... It's also more fun.... And easier on my body than trying to play a round of golf every day. These drills have changed the way I feel about putting."

She described the detail she applies in her practice. She divided the putt into two components – the distance and the line. "To putt well, one has to gauge the distance to the hole correctly as well as the line, the path the ball will take to the hole."

Here's how she described her line drill practice: "You set up six balls in a circle around the hole, two feet away. One by one, you putt them in. If you miss one, you start again. I usually practice this drill at the end of the day and I have to sink 25 in a row or I can't go home. The tension one feels when one has to make that 25th putt simulates the tension a golfer feels when she has to sink a putt to win a tournament." She's not done yet. She usually repeats the same drill with the balls three feet from the hole, trying to sink 25 in a row before going home. "You practice seeing the line of the putt and putting the ball on that line," she

---

10. K. Anders Ericsson, Ralf Th. Krampe, & Clemens Tesch-Romer, "The Role of Deliberate Practice in the Acquisition of Expert Performance," Psychological Review 100, 3 (1993), 363-406.

said. Eight weeks of deliberate practice like this helped her lower her handicap from 11 to 6.

Shelly Mars, a teaching tennis professional always gives her players the same advice, all of it related to focused practice: "If you don't focus, don't consider it practice", she says. "Don't just hit serves for an hour. Instead, consciously try to get 10 deep first serves in a row or reset and begin again." As a pro, she agrees: focus with practice is critical to improvement.

5: Remember – Mastery Takes Time

If we want to be good at something, *we have to give ourselves time.*

How good? How much time?

That depends. If you're already a busy professional, you may just want to be proficient at a sport. Or you may want to be good, in which case several years may be required. And what if you want to be *really* good – even world-class? Then it takes ten years, 10,000 hours of deliberate practice, says Dr. Ericsson. (That's about 19 hours a week and 2.7 hours a day for ten years.)

Directing 20-year studies of world-class performers in music, sports, mathematics, and chess, Dr. Ericsson has found that deliberate practice over ten years, 10,000 hours, determines excellence more than raw intelligence, talent, or concentrated but

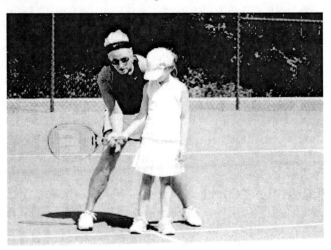

Shelly Mars teaching the forehand.
PHOTOGRAPH BY DEAN FORBES.

short bouts of hard work. In Ericsson's 20-year study of violinists, for example, the best group averaged 10,000 hours of deliberate practice, the next-best 7,500 hours, and the next 5,000 hours. My research on 103 national- and world-class masters runners generally supports Ericsson's theory.[11] It took them an average of eight and a half years to reach their best times, whether they started running in their youth or after age 30. So guess what. You are capable of doing anything and doing it well. Just *MOVE!*

But, you may say, it's too late, isn't it, to catch up with people who started when they were young? Not necessarily. Diane Hoffman, the tennis player who has won a world age-group championship and multiple national age-group championships, picked up a racket when she was 42 and was beating opponents 30 years younger in club tournaments when she was in her seventies. She was inducted into the US Tennis Association New England Hall of Fame at 83, almost 84. Sabra Harvey started running at 51 and discovered a talent, setting a world record in the half mile at 60 in 2:34.66, a time posted by some Division 3 college runners.

It is possible, moreover, after eight and a half years, for women who started running after 40 to run as fast as women who started running in their teens. A few late starters ran times seen in today's Division I college runners, if not the top runners. Times of late starters include a 5:08 mile for a 48-year-old and a 3:03 marathon for a 54-year-old.

The diagram on page 78 shows late starters "catching up" to the early starters.

You may not care about world class or even national class, but knowing that mastery takes time can be comforting. You've got time to make mistakes, learn from them, and come back. It also reminds you that <u>you are in control</u>. If you find an activity you are passionate about, you don't have to worry about lack of talent – something out of your control. You can succeed at levels you never thought possible. You can become a competitive tennis player, have a low golf handicap, win a rowing competition in the Paralympics (the major international multi-sport event for athletes with physical and visual disabilities), ski confidently,

---

11. Utzschneider, Women Runners.

run an eight or ten minute mile, finish an Iron Man or hike the Appalachian Trail. Depending on your circumstances, mastery could mean simply walking, running a mile or rowing the length of a competitive course untimed. It doesn't matter. Just remember, whatever level proficiency you are after, it takes time.

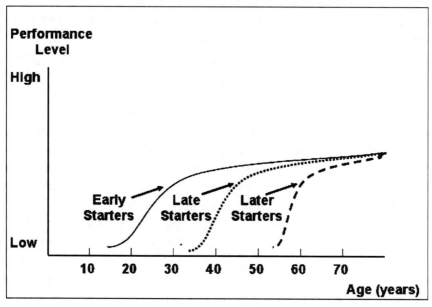

From: Utzschneider November 2007[12]

You may have such a full schedule with a family and career that you want to set a very long-term athletic goal – one you know will take decades, even a lifetime. That's the case with Dr. Irays Santamaria, a prosthodonist – a dentist who specializes in reconstructive and aesthetic dentistry – who came to this country from Venezuela to specialize in her field and open a private practice here. After ten years of graduate dental schooling, Dr. Santamaria now works 32 hours a week. She is also the mother of two children in elementary school. Her leisure time is limited, and she does have many interests – tennis, cooking, and piano among them.

Two years ago at 35, she took up tennis with her husband, also a dentist, and since then they've taken lessons every Friday

---

12. Ibid., p. 116-120.

morning throughout the year. On Sundays they play tennis with their children. "My goal is to be able to play a good game of doubles, though I am not sure that I will do it in a competitive way. I have many friends who do compete and they play really well and I would love to be able to play with them."

Mastery in the game of tennis in doubles, she said, may take her 30 years or more given her chosen schedule. "I have the rest of my life," she said. Tennis for her is "a long-term interest. One time we went to the tennis court and my daughter said 'that grandmother is really good!'. I love it when I see someone much older on the tennis court. That's who I want to be -- 75 and practicing sports in a safe and happy way."

PART II

The Practice

5 Implementing *MOVE!*

*"If you don't have a plan for yourself,
you'll be part of someone else's."*
- American Proverb

---

*Quick and easy forms allow you to track your progress and guide
you through the process. You don't have to use all of them.*

A buddy makes the adventure more fun.

A coach helps you focus your training and advance more quickly.

A weekly appointment with yourself reinforces commitment.

The Forms – Do I Really Need Them????

Forms remind me of taxes – do I really need them? I hate forms.

Yes, you need them.

As mentioned previously, the forms are a critical part of implementing the *MOVE!* method. The forms are simple and easy to complete and blank forms are available on my website, www.movegoals.com. The forms help you set, manage, review, and move to your next athletic goal. The forms give you perspective on where you are in the process. They also help you meet your goal faster, incorporate failure as part of learning and success (this is important), and confirm the path you've chosen while allowing flexibility and a change of course. Examples of completed forms appear throughout these chapters, while blank forms appear in the Appendix. Some of the forms are for planning, while others are for reviewing your achievements.

Don't forget: the forms are important to the process of achieving your goals. However, while all of the forms are valuable, you don't have to use all of them. Ultimately, the forms support the system, not vice versa.

The forms are the:

1) Athletic Options
2) Big Picture Calendar
3) Vision Statement
4) Short-Term Athletic Goal
5) Weekly Self Check-In
6) Buddy Discussion
7) Weekly Training Journal
8) Short-Term Goal Review
9) Annual Athletic Goal
10) Three Month Calendar
11) Overcoming Doubts and Fears
12) Post-Goal Analysis, and
13) Annual Goal Review.

The forms can be used for any sport. They are general enough so that you can tailor them successfully to your own non-athletic needs as well. You can use or adapt the forms for your professional or personal goals, tailoring some of them and using others in their original form. The forms help make your goals and passions real and objective. They help provide a record – a focused roadmap. When you complete the forms, you ensure commitment to your goals. Commitment to goals means achieving them.

In my Competitive Performance class one year, I didn't require students to submit training records along with their papers on athletic goals. That year only five of 16 students completed their goals. In other years, when they were required to submit training records, the percentage of goal achievement has ranged from 85 to 90%.

Records help you remember what you did two days ago and will help you evaluate your achievement when you're finished. Record keeping validates your efforts. Most importantly, if you experience pain or an injury during the process, the training journal gives you a place to record the pain or injury and track it on a scale of 1 to 5. With pain or an injury, you'll see whether the problem is increasing or decreasing, and be able to correlate it with what you're doing which will help you discover how to alleviate it.

For a training journal, any generic calendar that shows the days of the week and displays one week on a page suffices. You don't need a sports calendar, but you do need some kind of calendar to note progress. You can use the weekly training journal included here or you can create your own calendar by ordering one at www.personallogs.com. With a personally generated calendar, you can put your photo and name on the cover and even choose the journal start date.

How you fill out the training journal and the forms in general is up to you. You can write "bare bones" notes – or as much as you want. Say, you're a swimmer. You might just write: ¾ mile swim, the time it took, relevant strength and stretching exercises you did, what you'd eaten that day, the weather, your heart rate, and so forth. Or you can add details about your feelings or anything else you think is important.

The Buddy System

Why? As with filling out the forms and the training log, having a "buddy" – and the buddy system – is critical to *MOVE!* and therefore to achieving your goal. A buddy adds to the accountability and commitment to stick with the training process. A buddy provides a second opinion, support, and makes training week-to-week more fun. Indeed, it helps to improve training and helps make your goals more real.

Supporting these findings is a study conducted by Stanford University Professor of Health Research and Policy Abby King that found that social support in the form of a phone call plays a huge role in exercise.[13] Two hundred and eighteen people were divided into three groups and asked to walk half an hour most days of the week. (Government recommendations call for 150 minutes of walking in a week.) One group received a call every three weeks from a Stanford health educator who cheered them on and asked about their compliance. A second group received similar calls from a computer. A third group received no call at all. After 12 months, those who received a call from a live person increased their exercise from 100 to 178 minutes a week, a 78% jump. Those who received computerized calls doubled to 157 minutes a week. The third group that received no calls exercised 118 minutes a week, up 28% from the start of the study.

It is important to remember that you do not have to be a beginner to benefit from the accountability that another person provides. Wendy Wilbur used the *MOVE!* buddy system for some indoor rowing goals. Former World Champion, and seven-time U.S. national team member, Wilbur – who is now Coaching Assistant for Radcliffe Crew at Harvard University – affirms the value of the buddy system for small as well as large goals: "Being held accountable is something that is underrated. The thing that I

---

13. Abby C. King, Robert Friedman, Bess Marcus, Cynthia Castro, Melissa Napolitano, David Ahn, & Lawrence Baker, "Ongoing Physical Activity Advice by Humans Versus Computers: The Community Health Advice by Telephone (CHAT) Trial," Journal of Health Psychology 26:6 (2007), 718-727.

found is when you have somebody to check in with, even if you go off track for a couple of days, knowing that someone is depending on you gets you back on track. I don't want to let myself down or let my buddy down and say 'I didn't do anything this week'."

So, yes, personal support is important, but why a buddy if you already have support from a husband, partner, or others at home? Entrepreneur Leslie Kagan explains. "I didn't want to ask my husband for committed, sustained support for training," she said. "You don't want to overburden a relationship with too many expectations. At home you look to your partner/spouse for emotional support in a lot of domains. Your relationship goes through cycles of intimacy and availability and when you are taking on a major athletic event you don't want your support to be subject to that conditionality. I am a big believer that no one person should be expected to meet all of our emotional requirements. Having external support frees up your partner at home to be spontaneously enthusiastic without having to provide sustained emotional support."

When? You'll want to check in with your buddy once a week, at the same time every week for 5 to 15 minutes. Arrange an in-person, phone, or e-mail appointment.

Who can be your buddy? While it's best if that person is also pursuing a physical goal – it doesn't have to be the same or even the same kind as yours – an effective buddy can be anyone, whether or not he or she knows anything about your sport. The only requirement is that the person also be committed to your weekly meeting, understands you, your values, and your priorities, and wishes you the best and believes in your dreams. You may find your greatest supporters outside the athletic world. In fact, those outside could be the best supporters for you because they are objective about your situation.

Where? Where do you find a buddy if it's not at home or not in your sport? You can find emotional support anywhere if you know the warm feeling of being around it. You may find your buddy anywhere among your friends and acquaintances, in an athletic club, next door, at work, at church, in your book group. Anyone – again, as long as she/he believes in you, is committed to meeting with you and to encouraging you, both in your successes and your failures.

<u>What?</u> What should you be asking your prospective buddy? First, identify the kind of support you want. It can take different forms. Need a cheerleader? Someone to train with? Someone to watch your kids? Someone to help you say "no" to distractions? Someone to come to your event or give you a ride to your training site? A combination of these? Find a person who can and is 100% willing to fill your buddy needs.

<u>How?</u> What goes on during your buddy time? Here's one structure that works. Each person takes three minutes to talk, while the other person only listens. Then allot three minutes each to discuss possible solutions to any issues that have arisen. Remember, you're trying to make and sustain a change in your behavior. No change is easy, particularly when you're surrounded by distractions. Limit your buddy meeting to 15 minutes at the most. It's easy to digress.

Questions to discuss with your buddy might include: Why is this goal important? Should it be revised? What helped and what hurt your training this week? What are your greatest fears or obstacles? How can you anticipate and overcome them? Making a plan for the following week with your buddy is critical. You'll find the Buddy Discussion form in Chapter 6 and a completed copy in the Appendix.

Runners Leni Webber and Julie Burke not only talked each week but also trained together. They ran through three weeks of sub-zero temperatures training. "We were the only ones out there with face masks and nose warmers," said Leni. "We looked like the lone bandits. The buddy system got us out there."

Buddies Susan Smith and Martha Cole e-mailed each other each week, a golfer and tennis player respectively – both of them beginners. They wanted each other as buddies because they felt they needed mental strategies and support for competition. It didn't matter to them that one was focused on improving her drive and the other on improving her net game. "We both were trying to better our skills and also to learn how to stay relaxed when we were not playing well," said Martha. "The fact that we were in different sports and yet could relate to each other's issues was great. We knew we weren't competing with each other and that we wanted the best for each other."

"It didn't matter at all that we were in different sports," said Susan. "The competitive issues are universal, and talking to someone outside the golf or tennis circle helped bring an objective perspective to it."

Triathlete/runner Leslie Ouellette and runner Karen Shanley spoke once a week over the phone in preparation for Thanksgiving Day races. "We looked forward to reporting in every Wednesday evening for five or ten minutes," said Leslie...."

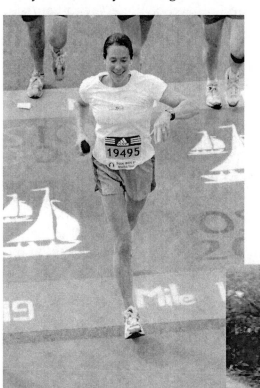

Leslie Ouellette, finishes the Boston Marathon. (right)

Karen Shanley on an early morning run. (below)

We both work and have kids –so we understand if one or other of us says "Do you mind if I make dinner while we talk?" "Of course not!"

"We didn't know each other well when we started doing this but have a lot in common," said Leslie. "Training has gotten better since I've gotten into the buddy system. It's a really fun experience… It's been great to hear each other's perspectives. People talk about kids giving unconditional love – this is unconditional support. The buddy system holds you to a different standard. There's no judgment; there's just support. You have your own support person. Accountability is the best part of the buddy system. You have to check in and be honest with yourself. You might cut corners on your own. Having a buddy makes your goals more real."

"It's been a wonderful source of support," said Karen. "We can give each other a 'second opinion' on what we're doing and that's so motivating. We are both committed to the process, and don't skip a week. It adds structure and fun to the whole training process. We talk not only about the details of training, but also about everything that affects it – work and family, sleep and nutrition, etc. It is great to have one person in your corner who listens to you about your training and whom you can also help. I tend to run too much and have a hard time cutting back. Leslie encourages me to cross train, particularly when I'm feeling tired. In fact, I'm at the gym right now, and I've just been on the elliptical machine!"

Buddies For Teams

You met Acacia Walker, a Boston College lacrosse coach and member of the World Cup Lacrosse Team, in Chapter 3. She used the Buddy System for the Boston College lacrosse team during a critical week in its season. The typical NCAA Division I season was over, and the team had a week before it heard whether it qualified for the finals.

During the wait-and-see week, we discussed how *MOVE!*

might help the team. "We were in a place where we couldn't stop all our bad habits," Acacia said. "We couldn't get the girls to improve in important areas."

In our talks, she commented that "girls are obsessed with keeping each other happy. Thirty percent of female athletes are real competitors, and seventy percent mark their success by how well liked they are by their teammates."

We discussed how the buddy system could use this motivation of wanting to be liked and of being team-oriented to reduce some of the girls' bad habits.

Girls were separated into buddy pairs. "Each girl had to identify two habits they wanted to work on. An ability to scoop ground balls is one of them." Instead of telling a player she had to sprint if she missed a ground ball – a standard motivational technique of coaches – Acacia used the psychology of the buddy system. She developed one variation whereby a player's error resulted in the buddy doing a sprint if she missed a ground ball.

"Because they are team-oriented and want to be liked, no one wanted to make their partner do an extra sprint," said Acacia. "All week long, they worked so hard because they didn't want their buddies to pay the consequences."

The result?

The players made fewer errors. "The buddy system of *MOVE!* is incredible," said Acacia. "It helped SO much. So much. These girls didn't want their teammates to do extra. That's how we started to get the girls to get rid of their bad habits."

Acacia found a way to use the fundamental principle of the Buddy System, that buddies support each other, to motivate the girls to perform better.

And the good news was that they made it into the tournament.

Do I Really Need A Coach Too?

Unlike a buddy, a coach, personal trainer, instructor, or someone – even a friend – whom you consider an expert in your sport provides you with guidance about skill development that a buddy without experience or expertise cannot. You should consult the person whom you consider an expert, your "coach", at least once every two weeks.

Experts can help you find your "baseline" – your level of competence or fitness in the activity you choose and help you set your goal. If you are focused on golf, for example, are you a novice or are you taking it up after many years of not playing? If so, what should you focus on first? You might go to a course and play with a pro. If you're a swimmer, how many laps can you swim in 10 minutes? A runner? How many minutes would it take to cover a mile? A rower? How long does it take to row 500 meters? And so on. A good coach will take those metrics and his or her knowledge of you to help you establish reasonable short- and long-term goals.

Depending on the sport, you may find an expert at fitness clubs, sports clubs, stores that specialize in your sport, local schools or colleges, community adult education programs, the Yellow Pages, and, of course, the internet. Obviously, you have to be careful, particularly if you are looking in the Yellow Pages or the internet. References are essential and need to be called. Three references are a minimum and you must, at least, talk on the phone with those making the references. If, for example, you are looking for a personal trainer, one of the best certifications is from the American College of Sports Medicine. If you want to swim a mile, you might want to consult your town recreation department for swim instructors. If you want to hike Mount Katahdin you might speak with an experienced hiker working at a sports store.

When you find a coach or trainer, you'll want to find out how he or she works with athletes. Can he or she help you set goals, define a weekly training program, and decide on equipment you'll need? If you don't think a particular coach fits, don't be hesitant. Try a new one until you get comments and a training program that suit you. Even if you have a coach who is not familiar with the *MOVE!* method, you can still use *MOVE!*.

Rower Jane Morse is enthusiastic about the benefit of coaching to accelerate progress versus acting on your own without expert advice. Without coaching, progress can take longer and bad habits can develop. Jane started rowing at 55 after a 30-year career in computer technology management that required long hours and so much traveling that rowing was not something she considered until she retired. In the beginning, she had no instruction and made no progress. Since then, she has always sought out a coach.

"Coaches push you," she said. "I've had a dozen coaches in the past decade. They have given me a training plan and terrific feedback on technique.

"Being coached makes you make changes. It provides some objectivity. A coach can help you make the changes that make you a better rower. When I started I didn't know anything about rowing or training. My coaches have provided me with the training program that made me strong."

The Weekly Appointment With Yourself

Setting aside just ten minutes for a weekly appointment with yourself helps you reflect on your goal (which can be adjusted), see where you are in the process, and gives you a chance to think "outside the box" and decide if you want to add and subtract aspects of your training. And yes, it *is* important to success. Note the time of your appointment just as you would an appointment with another person. Keep the appointment! If you miss it, impose a penalty on yourself such as agreeing to pay someone else a certain amount of money for every missed time.

During your appointment with yourself always ask the questions on the **Weekly Self Check-In** form (page 94). Answering questions such as "What was the plan for the past week and did you follow it?" and "Have you been too ambitious?" helps you adjust your goal if necessary and see whether you are on track.

Most of all, remember, your goals should be motivating, not defeating. Adjustment to the realities of life from time to time is OK. With *MOVE!*, flexibility is key. You will get to where you want to be eventually. Even with setbacks, you will achieve – and sometimes surprise yourself and even surpass your original goal. But a weekly self-assessment is important to properly gauge how you are doing and how you are feeling about the process.

Weekly Self Check-In -- Completed

Date: __March 5__

Week # : __3__

Have you written down what you did in the simplest terms? __Yes__

What was the plan for the past week and did you follow it? __All days__
__except for Monday – allergies bad.__

What is the plan for this week? __On three month training calendar__

If you got sick or encountered another obstacle, do you need to adjust
your goal date? __No__

How is your energy? __Fine except when pollen index really high.__

If you are not doing enough, what is holding you back? Are you doing
too much? Have you been too ambitious? Should you consider scaling
back your overall goal or adjust the time estimated to achieve it? Can
you adjust the smaller goals leaving the long-term goal intact?

__Ok so far. Not a problem.__

"You can't win them all -- but you can try." -Babe Didrikson

Preparing For and Setting Goals :
The Importance of
Writing Things Down

"Sweat and trust go together."
- Cathy Utzschneider

Preparing for goals before you set them is critical.

The Big Picture Calendar and Athletic Options form help you decide on goals that match your interests and schedule.

Having and writing down your vision is key to setting a goal.

The core of goal setting is the Short-Term Athletic Goal form. The Buddy Discussion form suggests questions for topics to talk about with your buddy.

You can set any of performance, outcome, or process goals.

The Three Month Training Calendar helps you visualize training for three months, which helps you see progression more clearly than a one-month calendar.

Ready to prepare for and set a goal?

Preparing For Goals

Preparing for goals is a critical though not lengthy phase in the *MOVE!* method. Literature related to goal setting does not always stress preparation before you set your goals, which includes consideration of what else is going on in the rest of your life. Preparing for goals is, in fact, a phase in goal achievement which many people don't even consider. They jump right into setting goals, the result being that they're not realistic. They're impractical given what else is going on in their lives. "I've never thought about preparing for goals," said Cyndy Cole, a school psychologist whom I met on a plane. "I never heard anybody say that!"

As mentioned before, the *first* step in preparing to set any physical goal is to receive approval from your physician that you are capable of physical activity. Next, develop a **Big Picture Calendar** (page 97). It helps you think of all the commitments in your life for the coming year. Chart major events on it – travel, anniversaries, school fairs, household projects, conferences. Seeing everything in one place will show where you have room – or where you can make room – for physical goals so you don't bump into unforeseen obstacles. Once you've identified your long-term athletic goal, note it on the Big Picture Calendar as a reminder of your future course.

Dr. Barbara Porter said that the big picture calendar exercise was helpful to her in itself because she didn't realize how many responsibilities she was juggling before she started rowing. "I didn't realize how many professional and personal commitments I already had – and I had to get my professional and personal life in order so that I had time for rowing," she said. "If you want to be successful with a goal, you really have to look ahead before adding something in. You have to consider not only your schedule but also your husband's, and your family's schedules too."

In addition, review your weekly schedule. When do you

Big Picture Calendar -- Completed

Responsibilities	January	February	March	April	May	June
Family/Friends			Leahey Wedding			
Personal	45th Birthday!					
Work				Conference		
Home	Mortgage					Refinancing
Athletic			10K Road Race			

"Just go out there and do what you've got to do." –Martina Navratilova

Big Picture Calendar -- Completed

Responsibilities	July	August	September	October	November	December
Family/ Friends			Rick–Toronto		Thanksgiving	Christmas
Personal						Vermont Trip
Work						
Home				House Painting		
Athletic		10K Road Race				

"Just go out there and do what you've got to do." - Martina Navratilova

Big Picture Calendar -- Completed

1. What is my long-term goal?

Earn an age-graded 10k time which beats my best time from cross country in college.

2. How will the commitments listed above affect my pursuit of that goal?

I will schedule my races around the commitments in other areas of my life so I'll be able to give 100% of my focus to my race. I don't want to race tired!

3. How will I handle "distractions" so they're compatible with my life as a whole?

Acknowledge that things come up that will "sidetrack" me. Remember to look at all these commitments and try to keep others to a minimum so I can focus on my main goals.

"Just go out there and do what you've got to do." –Martina Navratilova

really have free time? Be careful to allow transition time between activities.

After completing a Big Picture Calendar and getting a handle on your weekly schedule, the next step if you're not sure what sport you want to pursue is the **Athletic Options** form (page 101). It asks you to list the various activities you are considering and possible goals you'd like to achieve within a year. Review all the pros and cons of each sport: How many hours does the sport require for one session from start to finish? What fits into your schedule? Are you more interested in cardiovascular fitness, competitive achievement, skill development, or weight loss? Consider all pertinent logistics including access to training places (pools, tracks, tennis or squash courts, for example) equipment needed, coaching availability, etc., and club memberships. Choose the activity with the most "pros". Promise yourself you'll try your sport by a particular date. Starting anything new is a big step so give yourself credit for experimenting.

The Athletic Options form helps you choose a sport that's realistic given your circumstances. "I've always wanted to learn to ride a bike. Believe it or not, I've never had one," said Leslie Lewis, 32 and a mother of three. "I grew up in New York City and in school did ballet but otherwise was not sporty." The Athletic Options form helped her figure out all relevant logistics ahead of time – including where she would buy a bike, when she would need a baby sitter, and which routes to ride. "Just thinking through all the details helped me start my goal more smoothly," she said.

As you experiment with possible athletic activities, think for yourself and listen to your feelings. Do you want to compete? Do you prefer a group or individual activity? If I were at the end of my life, what would I want to have done? What am I afraid of but also drawn to? If you're not sure what to do, jot down ideas daily in a notebook. If the same thoughts emerge day after day, in time you'll see a pattern pointing towards your athletic goal.

"When you feel a pull, follow it," said hiker Cheryl Suchors, whose experiment led to hiking 48 mountains over 4,000 feet in New Hampshire. "Find a way to follow that thing that makes your face light up.

Athletic Options -- Completed

1. List the various athletic or other activities you are considering:

    A. _Yoga_

    B. _Skiing_

    C. _Hiking_

    D. _Swimming_

2. Number of hours per week, including travel time, for your sport given other life commitments (family, household, work, community, etc.)

6-7 hours a week

3. Specify hours you can exercise each day, including travel time:

Mon: _6-8 a.m._ Tues: _zip_ Weds: _6-8 a.m._ Thurs: _zero_
Fri: _6-8 a.m._ Sat: _depends_ Sun: _10 to noon_

4. What do you want from a sport (note top, middle, and bottom priority with a 1, 2, and 3 respectively)?

Cardiovascular fitness _1_ Strength _3_ Skill _3_ Friendship _1_
Mental challenge _2_ Competitive achievement _3_ Weight loss _1_
Decreased stress _1_ Cessation of bad habits (smoking, overeating, etc.) _2_ Stronger relationship with partner _3_

5. List the pros and cons of each sport or activity option:

Sport: _Yoga_

Pros: _I need quiet time in my life. I need to build strength_

and flexibility.

"It is better to look ahead and prepare than to look back and regret" -Jackie Joyner Kersee

Athletic Options -- Completed

Cons: _I need more cardiovascular exercise and I want to train outdoors sometimes._

Sport: _Skiing_

Pros: _It's a family sport. I love the feeling of skiing._

Cons: _Pricey and seasonal. Should buy all new equipment._

Sport: _Swimming_

Pros: _I want to do the Swim Against the Tide for Mom. I'll get in cardiovascular shape and get strong. I could work on the freestyle technique which would be fun. Can swim indoors in the winter and outdoors on the lake in the summer._

Cons: _The black line at the bottom of the pool doesn't talk to me._

6. Special logistics to consider for each sport:

Outside care: _Need to get care for Dad._

Pet care: _OK in crate for a few hours._

Equipment needed: _Swimming – minimal – suit/goggles; hiking minimal – have boots, warm clothes. Skiing – need new equipment – expensive. Yoga – minimal. Mat._

"It is better to look ahead and prepare than to look back and regret" -Jackie Joyner Kersee

Athletic Options -- Completed

Coach available: _Not sure. Depends. Yoga, yes. Skiing yes._

Hiking? Consult masters swim coach ?

Place to train needed: _None - town has good pool and times_

reserved for swimmers fit my schedule.

Others to train with: _Frank? Both game for all but yoga._

Hours of travel required: _Swimming, yoga — minimal; hiking,_

skiing — 90 min. for sport. Minimal for dialing training.

7. Based on the pros and cons above, what's it going to be?

Swimming.

8. Consult with a doctor about your choice. _Done._

9. Make a commitment to try your sport on a particular day and try it three times.

"It is better to look ahead and prepare than to look back and regret" -Jackie Joyner Kersee

"When I first heard about the 4,000 Footer club, it just moved me," said Cheryl. "It wasn't because someone else was doing it. It would get me out into nature and I could do it on my own terms in my own way. I liked the freedom to decide when I hiked and whether I would hike by myself, with my husband, friends, or family. I was interested in learning about equipment, technique, camping, lightning, wild flowers, and about how to read weather and maps.... I wanted to learn about toads and birds because I was going into their environment."

Use common sense to judge how long you experiment – but give the athletic activity a chance. Are you someone who doesn't enjoy something until you're very comfortable with it? You can experiment with running more easily and quickly than you can with scuba diving but it's important with something like running not to go out of the box too quickly. Injury or frustration can result if you are too aggressive in your goals. Sometimes the easiest isn't the best. Again, always enter the "beginner's mind".

Remember, it's OK to realize the sport you initially chose is not the one for you. Try another sport. How long you should experiment with a sport will depend on your sport, your desires, your personality, and your previous background or level of experience in that sport or a related one. A reasonable experiment is to try out your sport three times before you dismiss it. Of course some sports like scuba diving require a longer initial commitment. Experiment long enough to know whether or not you're motivated and ready to set a short-term goal.

Once you've taken the time to think about your whole life and a sport that fits with your schedule, you're ready to set a goal.

Setting Goals Begins With The Vision Statement

What do I mean by "vision" – and why start setting a goal with one?

A vision describes how you want to perform, look, or feel when you achieve your final goal; it helps you create a mental picture of your target. As with goals, it is important to write down your vision. That vision becomes your "vision statement".

A **Vision Statement** (page 106) helps support your long-term dream. For novice and Olympic athletes alike – belief in ourselves can be a challenge. We can be our own worst critics. It's been said that athletes' physical potential is twelve times greater than they think.

You might say, *"But I'm not sure I really have a vision yet! The thought of me as accomplished in a new sport seems absurd, not to mention unrealistic."* The point is that this vision is exactly what is going to motivate you out the door for your day-to-day training. Images are powerful – "a picture is worth a thousand words." While you may think yours is unrealistic or impossible to live up to at the moment, if you give yourself enough time, it can become reality. I've seen many athletes look back on their vision statements, amazed that they realized them.

This motto on the vision statement form says it all: "Dream it. Speak it. Believe it. Do it." Describe your vision statement in the present tense as if you are reporting what you actually see, hear, think, and feel.

My suggestion is to type and frame your vision statement to make it real and permanent. Short, concise statements are more effective than long ones because they are easier to remember (two sentences at most). Put it in a place (bathroom mirror or refrigerator, for example) where you can see and think about it every day.

A vision statement can also be a picture of an athlete you wish to emulate. Tennis player Linda used an image, rather than a statement, to support her long-term goal of winning a Singles "A" level championship. "I found a picture of Chris Evert when she was young," she said. "I have always admired her cool demeanor and just her picture reminded me of my goal of remaining emotionally detached during matches. The picture was more powerful than any words because it captured so many additional traits I wanted to have as a tennis player. I wanted smooth strokes. Anyway, I put the photo of Chris on my desk and it moved into my subconscious. I thought about having her cool grace when I sat at my desk – and when I stepped on the court."

Vision Statement -- Completed

Dream it. Speak it. Write it. Believe it.

Type and frame your vision statement to make it real and permanent. Short, concise statements are more effective than long ones because they are easier to remember (two sentences at most). Put it in a place (bedside table or other) where you can see and think about it every day.

Athletes have vision. *What's yours?*

------------------------------------CUT HERE---

My vision: <u>I am a competent doubles player. I rush the net</u>

<u>after serving and feel confident before each point no matter</u>

<u>how the last one went.</u>

Now we should discuss the specifics of setting the actual goals themselves. Ideally, the goal you set for yourself should be a combination of performance, outcome, and process goals. Here's what each goal means.

Performance, Outcome, And Process Goals

A *performance goal* is the end result that you, personally, want to achieve – a standard of accomplishment that is independent of other athletes' performances. Some examples:

- I will walk a mile in 25 minutes.
- I will raise my tennis game from a 3.0 to a 3.5 level.
- I will perfect my crawl so I can swim 10 consecutive laps.
- I will bike 25 miles in 2:00 to 2:15 hours.
- I will hike Mount Washington in 7.5 to 8 hours, including ascent and descent.

An outcome goal is a goal relative to other athletes' performances. Outcome goals are goals of competition, whether direct or indirect. People experienced in a sport are more likely than beginners to set an outcome goal. Performance goals generally have a higher ratio of success than outcome goals because you have more control over them. You don't have control over someone else's performance. Some examples of outcome goals are:

- I will challenge my husband Tom to see who can walk a mile faster.
- I will reach at least the quarterfinals of the club tennis tournament.
- I will challenge my friend Mary to see who can swim 10 consecutive laps faster.
- I will finish this 25 mile ride in the top 10% of women in my age group.
- I will hike Mount Washington faster than my brother did (he completed the hike in 7 ¼ hours).

Whether or not you choose to set a performance or an

107

outcome goal, *process goals are essential*. A process goal is a specific training task that you will perform on a weekly basis. Some experts use the term "process goal" and "task goal" interchangeably. A process goal may include cardiovascular training as well as intensity, strength, flexibility, mental or skill training. A nutritional process goal might be to drink 64 ounces of water a day.

The more focused your process goals, the more you can incorporate deliberate practice, a key to excellence discussed in Chapter 4. Your process goals should include practice that is repeated consistently, that target your weaknesses and specific needs, and that can be adjusted regularly based on feedback from a coach. Setting your process goals in terms of ranges ("I will do 25 sit-ups three to five times a week") allows for some variability and ensures success.

Process goals tend to be more detailed the more advanced you are. A weekly process goal for a beginner-level runner might be to incorporate 30 second jogs in 30 minutes of walking four to six times a week and to stretch for ten to 15 minutes five times a week.

A process goal for an elite middle distance runner may be more complex. It might be to run 50 to 60 miles a week, incorporating between six to eight miles of threshold running (running at about 80% of maximum effort) and four miles of intervals at 90% of maximum effort; strength train two to three times a week for 25 to 35 minutes at a time; stretch for 15 to 20 minutes five to six times a week; practice yoga once or twice a week; visualize the third quarter of the 10K race for at least five minutes three times a week; take a multiple vitamin with iron daily; drink the equivalent of 10 to 12 glasses of water daily; and eat at least five to six fruits a day.

A coach or someone more experienced can help you identify and set performance, outcome, and process goals.

Short-Term Athletic Goals

Having established your vision and decided on your type of goal, you're ready to set a short-term goal that is the core of the *MOVE!* method. The **Short-Term Athletic Goal** form (page 110) is so basic that it can be tailored to any sport. If you don't find all categories applicable, leave them blank and add some of your own. Make your first short-term athletic goal just six weeks long, and make it a modest goal – even more modest than you think is reasonable at first. You can make short-term goals more challenging later.

Now is also the time to find a coach, instructor, or someone experienced in your chosen sport to discuss your long-term athletic goal. Once you've set up a training relationship, have that person assess for themselves your current level of proficiency or baseline. Discuss your baseline, your assessment of your current level of competence and theirs. Preferably, they will match but if they don't, that can also be good. It should lead to a discussion that could reveal much about each other's perspectives, your coach's coaching style and how it fits with you. You can also work with a coach or instructor on adjusting the Short-Term Athletic Goal form that will help both of you think realistically about your plan. What are your beginning and end dates? How would you now describe your baseline – your current level of competence – in the sport in light of your discussions?

The Buddy Discussion

It is also the time to look around for someone who might be a buddy – someone who can meet you, speak with you, Skype, or at least e-mail once a week at a specific time. All you need, if you are pressed for time, is just about twenty minutes to allow ten minutes for each of you to relate the week's progress and challenges, and to discuss questions and plans for the upcoming week. **The Buddy Discussion** form (page 112) suggests that you not only review your short-term athletic goal each week but also take notes on your buddy's weekly goals to ensure mutual accountability. The "meeting" with your buddy provides a chance to address all kinds of fears and possible solutions or ways to address them.

Short-Term Athletic Goal -- Completed

Goal: _Run 30 minutes with 2 one-minute walking breaks in the middle._

Current level: _Can jog for two minutes at a time. Then I need to walk. I can do 25 knee push-ups and 50 sit-ups (with effort)._

Beginning Date: _July 1st, 2011_

Ending Date: _August 12th, 2011_

# of weeks: _6_

Process Goals (Identify times per week)

Cardiovascular training: _Run/walk five days a week for 25 to 30 minutes 3 xs /week and 35 to 40 mins 2 xs/week. Start by alternating 2 mins. of jogging and 1 of walking._

Intensity: _None yet._

Strength: _25 to 30 push-ups and 50 to 70 sit-ups 3-4 xs/ week._

Flexibility: _10 to 15 minutes after each run._

Mental (reading, meditations, vision statements, etc.): _Daily mantra: "One step at a time."_

Skill development: _Get Cathy's comments on form._

"We can do anything we want as long as we stick to it long enough." - Helen Keller

Short-Term Athletic Goal -- Completed

Nutrition: _Take daily multi-vitamin. Drink 64 oz water daily. Only buy flavors of ice cream that I don't like._

Other (Balance, coordination): _Get workout clothes that make me feel serious (also new sneakers). Don't go overboard, though._

Challenges ahead:

1. _Keep training during family vacation._
2. _Run early in the a.m. during really hot days._

NON-ATHLETIC GOALS

1. _Write my blog every Friday from 9 to 10 a.m._
2. _"Pleasure "read for at least an hour a day._

OPTIONS FOR BUDDY

1. _Lisa_
2. _Martha_
3. _Joanne_

"We can do anything we want as long as we stick to it long enough." - Helen Keller

Buddy Discussion -- Completed

Topics for discussions/issues regarding Short-Term Goal Form and Training Journal:

1. Are your goals still realistic given your other commitments?

Yes — there may be conflict with school pick-up, occasionally.

2. What are your greatest fears (hot weather, doubts, etc.)?

I lose motivation after the first week.

3. How can you overcome those fears?

I will speak with buddy and get reinspired. I will also ask family for support. Take it slow.

4. Discuss training records and your weekly training journal.

5. Other.

Discuss and record solutions to your issues.

1. Build occasional school pick-up into training routine. Consider it a rest day or do short, intense workout but make it count, not interrupt training.

2. Call Martha when not motivated to train.

3. Practice riding with new clipless pedals in school parking lot.

"No one changes the world who isn't obsessed." -Billie Jean King

Buddy Discussion -- Completed

Action Plan:

I will meet with Martha three times a month to bike with the Charles River Wheelman. For the next two months (May and June) we will e-mail or call each other once a week on Thursdays at 8:00 p.m. to review training. If one of us misses a session we have to pay the other person $10! After two months we'll review this to see how we're doing, whether to revise this plan etc.

"No one changes the world who isn't obsessed." -Billie Jean King

The Weekly Training Journal

The **Weekly Training Journal** (page 115) to which we referred in the last chapter is critical to following your process goals and your overall progress or your short-term goal. Every week when you take a few minutes to review your training, you can check that you're on track or revise your short-term goal if you realize you were overly ambitious or not ambitious enough. Successive short-term athletic goals allow you to adjust them continually, leading to a long-term goal. What if, at the end of the six weeks, you haven't yet reached your goal? Easy. Extend the goal period by a few weeks. Again, goals are and should be reasonably flexible. They should be motivating, not defeating.

Longer Term Planning

The Three Month Training Calendar. Another important aspect of the process involves keeping a **Three Month Training Calendar** (page 116). This is helpful for planning and/or recording training so you can both plan for and track your progress over several months.

The Annual Athletic Goal. The **Annual Athletic Goal** form (page 119) that facilitates setting your long-term plan or goal is helpful *once you have completed at least one short-term goal.* If you don't care about a long-term goal, you can try another short-term goal. The experience of going for a short-term athletic goal will help you figure out your long-term goal with a more realistic and objective perspective. You will have already learned whether you tend to set your goals too high or not high enough. You will know what the obstacles are, and how much you really want to take on. You will know what motivates you.

The Annual Athletic Goal form is different from the Short-Term Goal form in that it simply reinforces the big picture and your commitment to a major goal as you set successive short-term

Weekly Training Journal -- Completed

Weekly Training	
Short-term physical goal: _Move up the tennis ladder to #15_	
Start Date: _June 1st, 2011_	
Finish Date: _July 15th, 2011_	

RECORD FOR WEEK # __1__	
Goals for week? Play 4 full matches. Focus on "Deliberate Practice". Fitness/agility training.	
Monday	Volleyed. Served.
Tuesday	Match 6-4, 3-5...ran out of time
Wednesday	After match, realize backhand needs to be deeper in court. 30 minutes just on backhands. 15 mins. volleys , 15 mins serves.
Thursday	Agility drills (jump rope and ladder hops) for 10 minutes. Court sprints for 10 minutes. Relaxed hitting for 30 minutes.
Friday	Match 6-2, 6-1
Saturday	Match 4-6, 6-2, 6-7 (3-7)
Sunday	Jog for 25 minutes

Not accomplished in weekly goal:

Played three, not four matches.

"God gives talent. Work transforms talent into genius." -Anna Pavlova

Three Month Training Calendar -- Completed

Year: 2011   Month: July

Monday	Tuesday	Wednesday	Thursday	Friday	Saturday	Sunday	Week Totals
rest	tempo run, 4mi.	easy 3-4	easy 4-5	easy 4	easy 2	5-6 easy	22-25 miles
rest	5-6 hills w/in 6	easy 3-4	easy 5-6	4 mi. w/ 6 strides	easy 3	easy 6-7	25-28
rest	4-5 X 800, 5 total	easy 4	easy 5-6	easy 5	easy 2	easy 2	28 - 30
easy 3	5-6 hill w/in 5	easy 4-5	easy 5 w/ strides	easy 5	rest	race 5k, 6-7 total	28 - 30
rest	4 X 1000, 5 total	easy 5					

"True champions aren't always the ones that win, but those with the most guts." -Mia Hamm

Three Month Training Calendar -- Completed

Year: 2011 **Month: August**

Monday	Tuesday	Wednesday	Thursday	Friday	Saturday	Sunday	Week Totals
rest	tempo run, 5 mi.		easy 5	easy 4	easy 4	7-9 easy	30-32
rest	3 X 1 mile, 6 total	easy 4-5	easy 6	6 hills, 4 mi.	easy 4	8-9 easy	32-34
		easy 5-6	easy 6	8 X 1 min., 5 mi.	easy 4	8 - 10 easy	34-37
easy 5	tempo run, 6 mi.	easy 7-8	easy 5 w/ 6 strides	easy 4	rest	race 5mi. or 10k	32-35
rest	6-7 hills, 5 mi.	easy 7-8	easy 5	5 mi. w/ 8 strides	easy 4		

"True champions aren't always the ones that win, but those with the most guts." –Mia Hamm

Three Month Training Calendar -- Completed

Year: 2011			Month: September					
Monday	Tuesday	Wednesday	Thursday	Friday	Saturday	Sunday	Week Totals
rest	6 – 7 X 800, 6 mi.	easy 7-8	easy 6	6 X 2 mins., 6 mi.	5 easy	8-10 easy	34-38
rest	5 X 600, 6 mi.	easy 6-7	easy 6	30 min. tempo, 7 mi.	4 easy	8-10 easy	38-42
rest	10 X 400, 6 mi	easy 4-5	easy 6	30 min. tempo, 7 mi.	4 easy	9-12 easy	38-42
						7-8 easy	35-37
easy 4	5 mi. w/ 8 strides	easy 5	easy 4	easy 3	rest	10k race	19-20 plus race

Annual Athletic Goal -- Completed

Beginning Date: _November 10th, 2011_
Ending Date: _November 10th, 2012_

MAIN ATHLETIC GOALS:

1. _Complete the Sturbridge to Bourne Ride (111 miles of the Pan Mass Challenge)._

2. _Run the Tufts 10K._

OTHER COMMITMENTS:

1. _Work — increase consulting business by 15% this year_

2. _Research and decide on assisted living facilities for Mom — finish by September._

3. _Enforce homework routine for kids (7-9 p.m.)_

4. _Join book club._

"Racing teaches us to challenge ourselves. It teaches us to push beyond where we thought we could go." -Patti Sue Plummer

athletic goals. The Annual Athletic Goal form guides you in setting your short-term goals. It asks you to list the main goals in the other areas of your life. They are affected by training and vice-versa. Like the Short-Term Goal form, the Annual Goal form asks for the beginning and ending date as well as your baseline – your level of fitness or skill at the start of your goal.

As the completed Annual Athletic Goal form shows, the runner's main goals in her other areas of life included increasing her consulting revenues by 15 percent, researching and deciding on assisted living facilities for an aging parent, and establishing a homework routine for her children. Knowing these major objectives in the other parts of her life helped her focus on her athletic goal both to accommodate it from a time perspective (i.e.

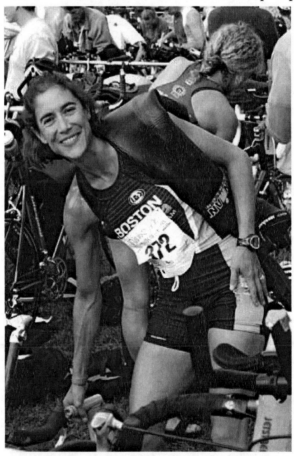

Sarah Keller during a transition in a Half Ironman.

busy schedule) but also in scheduling time for herself for her own physical and emotional health.

Professor of communications at Montana State University Billings, Sarah Keller discussed the benefits of setting long-term goals along with short-term goals. She juggles a lot – her career, a family, including two children, but also training for and competing in triathlons, and road races. Her goals have spanned years and have required a lot of forethought about other aspects of life as well as training. She could not, for example, plan her athletic goals without working around both her family and teaching.

"Setting long-term goals helps you understand where you are along the way. It's an opportunity to dream high and to articulate those dreams – which can be hard in itself. If you don't dream high, you don't get there. An advantage of setting other life goals with athletic goals is that you don't put all your eggs in one basket.

"If your entire being is wrapped up in one endeavor, it can be very painful when you have setbacks. It's always a rocky road to success. If you have aims other than physical goals in your life, it creates an opportunity for feeling good about yourself in another arena."

Setting goals helps you see not only what you can achieve, but also what you can't achieve realistically at given points in your life. It also helps you prioritize and, I hope, see the importance of setting an athletic goal – whatever it may be – for your own health and happiness.

Managing Goals: Doubts and Fears

*"Those who believe they can and
those who believe they can't are both right."*
- Anonymous

We have all kinds of doubts. Common ones include:

1. *I'm totally out of shape!*
2. *I'll get injured.*
3. *I have a physical limitation.*
4. *I'm too old.*
5. *It's too late to learn something new.*
6. *I've excelled at sports— I don't have the patience to be a beginner again.*
7. *I hate competition.*
8. *I'm too busy.*
9. *Getting started feels overwhelming.*

The Overcoming Doubts and Fears form can help you dismiss doubts.

So, you're starting to get excited about achieving that athletic goal you've dreamed about and you are beginning to think "Wow!" and then comes the …

"But ………!"

That's a word I'm familiar with. I hear women say that word a lot. Self-proclaimed non-athletes, former college athletes, even professional athletes express doubts. We *all* have doubts. At the thought of actually setting a new goal some laugh at themselves. Some shake their heads or roll their eyes. Some come up with a hundred excuses why now would be a difficult time. But – there's the word again – they're tempted and interested….and they're in my office for a reason.

Sorting out doubts is the first step in moving forward toward realizing your goal. Figure out which doubts are real and which are imagined. Then work around those that are real and deflate those that are imagined.

"I don't have doubts," you may say. If so, skip this chapter. But ask yourself if you are really being honest. Doubts not felt at the beginning can also crop up later.

So, if you do have doubts, this chapter covers several of the more common ones: various "physical" doubts about your body, and "biographical" doubts – questions about your ability to train in the context of the rest of life.

Physical Doubts

Doubt #1: I'm too fat and out of shape. If you're heavier than you would like, you're one of more than half of the adult American female population, if you look at recent statistics. More than 29 percent of women in the United States are overweight and an additional 24 percent are obese. *But you're never too heavy to set an athletic goal.* Needless to say, you'll need to start small (like everyone), build slowly, be patient, and consult with your physician.

Pam Kunkemueller didn't lose weight before setting her athletic goal. A grandmother in her late fifties at the time she started, she had 30 pounds to lose. She had a hard time walking up stairs. She started walking 20 to 25 minutes a day but to her astonishment after eight weeks she was exercising on her Nordic track for 40 to 45 minutes five times a week. A few years later she was jogging a few miles several times a week. She lost 16 pounds and her knee problems disappeared.

<u>Doubt #2: I'll get injured.</u>   There are risks with any new venture. Women over 40 should be particularly careful of injuries, but you can always minimize injures if you recognize them early enough. Back off immediately, and adopt a mentally flexible attitude. In the meantime, find other activities that don't aggravate the injury. Major successes can be enjoyed later.

If you don't risk, you don't succeed. Here are examples of success after injury. At age 54, runner Leni Webber incurred a groin injury. It stayed with her for a year and a half. She couldn't run. She swam, ran in the water, and biked on a recumbent bike. A year and a half later she resumed running, pain free, and trained for the most competitive event of her life: the Outdoor National Masters Track and Field Championships. She was in the shape of her life, having lost the five pounds she'd been trying to lose for ten years, and she won a bronze medal in her age group.

Even with an injury, there are ways around it. Madeline Pearlmutter has been skiing consistently since her late twenties despite having torn her anterior cruciate ligament (a knee ligament) in her forties, a tear that resulted from a summertime accident. Surgery was unsuccessful, but with physical therapy and training with weights twice a week to build the muscles around the knee, Madeline still downhill skis most weekends during the winter with a brace to support her knee. "Why not ski?" is Madeline's attitude. Her husband and children ski and, as long as she can enjoy recreational skiing, she will. "I love being outdoors in the winter and it's social," she said.

And what about chronic injuries like Achilles tendonitis that you may have incurred over decades of activity? Scientists are learning more and more new techniques to heal scar tissue. According to Dr. Joanne Borg-Stein, Medical Director of the Spaulding-Wellesley Rehabilitation Center, platelet-rich plasma therapy is one of them. It uses growth factors concentrated in the athlete's own platelets through a special process after which the platelets are then injected into the injured area with musculoskeletal ultrasound image guidance. This begins a new reparative process to heal chronic injury to tendons, ligaments, muscle and joints. So, never say never. It's always worth researching the latest improvements in medical treatments.

Doubt #3: I'm disabled, have a severe physical limitation or medical condition. More doubts of this kind can include: I have cancer, the medications I take make me really tired, I'm happy just appreciating the little things in life, taking up a new sport will be difficult.... I guess you're not writing this book for me! Thanks, but no thanks.

As I said in the beginning of this book, *MOVE!* is for everyone. Any athletic goal is possible if you think creatively and work around (or against) your disability. Many of us do have significant health issues – and they clearly vary in nature and severity. It is important to remember that an athletic goal does not have to be running the Boston Marathon, swimming a half mile or more every day or playing six sets of tennis. You may not be able to run, for example, if you have had a hip replacement or swim if you have shoulder problems... or play tennis well if you have arthritic elbows. You have to accept and work with your limitations or your condition.

Doubts – particularly about medical conditions – are ones to work around, not drown out. Listen, very respectfully, to your body. If you have an illness or are taking medications that cause fatigue, anemia, excessive sweating, whatever – by all means pay attention to it. An illness or painful condition may mean it's not the right time to pursue an athletic goal. On the other hand, maybe it is. Why cheat yourself out of what could be one of life's best surprises? If you think it's possible and have an interest in pursuing an athletic goal, the first step, of course, is to consult your physician. What can and can't you do? Many people who have trained through all kinds of illnesses have appreciated the *MOVE!* method and achieved their goals because it gave them something positive on which to focus.

Nancy Schuder is an example of one of many who worked around her disability. Nancy, 56, has a degenerative bone disease. As a result, she has had three surgeries on her left ankle. A rod inserted in it prevented any flexing. She cannot run, for example. In February of 2009, three months after her third ankle surgery, she had healed enough to start walking. In the first month, walking across her bedroom once a day was a painful accomplishment. In April, she decided on a three-month goal of biking three miles

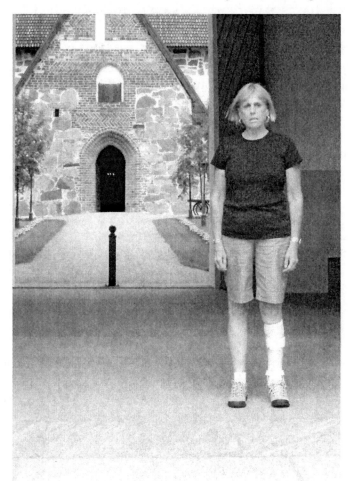

A walking goal was key to Nancy Schuder's recovery

and losing 20 pounds. She would limit her caloric intake to 1600 calories, lift upper body weights, swim, and begin to bike – three minutes at a time. She picked biking because she wanted to challenge her beliefs about the limitations of her ankle.

Three months later, Nancy achieved her biking goal and lost 25 pounds, five more than planned. She travelled to Europe and easily walked three or more miles a day without pain. Did she ever expect she would do this? "Absolutely not," she said. "I became so involved in the day-to-day process of training that I was thinking more about the process. I'd say, 'Today, this is what I need to do'. The goal was there in the background the whole time...but I was surprised, let's say amazed, when I actually reached the goal."

Remember also the story of Karin Miller who developed a crippling joint disease and turned to martial arts both as therapy and as a way to stay active. She now lives a "pain-free life". While this won't work for every disability, clearly you can achieve athletic goals and change your "mind-body connection", as she put it.

The motto here is never say "no". Challenge limiting beliefs. If one activity doesn't work for you, try another. Don't say you can't until you've tried everything.

Doubt #4: My body's too old for this.   It's too late. Your neurons aren't firing the way they used to. Your reactions are slower. It is true that at a certain age between the mid-twenties and age about 30, our bodies start to decline. Our capacity to do aerobic work declines by about 1% per year or 10% per decade. Flexibility, muscular strength, power, and reaction times decline also. You reach maximum muscular strength at about 25. By the time you're 70, you have 30% less overall strength if exercise is held constant. So...if you could bench press 150 pounds at 25, you can press 105 pounds at 70 even if you bench pressed regularly for the 45 intervening years.

If you're going to listen to the voice that tells you you're too old, you'll make your bed, lie in it, and never get up. Biological decline does occur at generally predictable rates. Cardiovascular capacity can be negatively affected by declining muscle volume, excess body fat, and illness – and while it's also determined by your genes – training both in terms of volume and intensity can improve it. As mentioned in the introduction, *your body is never too old to improve.* Studies have shown that, whereas the typical cardiovascular decline in inactive adults is about 10% per decade, men and women who continue training, incorporating intensity as well as endurance, can reduce cardiovascular decline from 10%

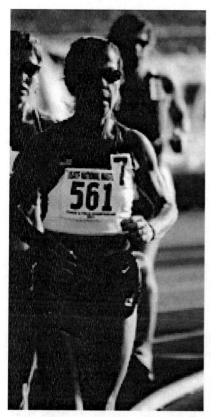

Kathy Martin racing at the World Masters Athletics Championships.
PHOTOGRAPH BY
GREGORY L. COATS SR.

to only 5% per decade.[14]

Consider athletic superstars who took up their sport in adult life while leading normal lives with careers, families, etc. Outstanding among masters women runners is Kathy Martin, now 60 – a realtor, wife, mother, and grandmother. She started running at about 30, and her world started to change: "I did not love running for the first 30 days," she said. "Each day, I would run one more mailbox or one more telephone pole, etc. And when I started doing speed, I always thought about the ice cream waiting for me at the end. I had to have the carrot there," she said. A five-mile race was her first distance race. "I loved racing immediately!" she said. " I never knew I had a competitive side until I started running!".

One of the most successful, "winning-est" masters runners in the world, Martin has run times in her fifties that would qualify her for a Division 1 college track and cross country team. Some of her running times improved not just through her thirties but through her forties and even into her fifties. For example, while she ran a terrific 10K time when she was 34 – a time of 36:54 – she ran her fastest 10K time ever at 51 in 36:31. At 52, she was featured running in a Nike television commercial. Martin expresses it best: "Yahoo for aging!"

---

14. Scott W. Trappe, David L. Costill, Matthew D. Vukovich, James Jones, & Thomas Melham, "Aging Among Elite Distance Runners: a 22-Year Longitudinal Study" Journal of Applied Physiology 80:1 (1996), 285-290.

True, Martin is a phenom. Yet there are other masters runners over 40 – and masters athletes in other sports – who can challenge and, on a given day, beat 20-year-olds.

Who knows what you can do? The potential of the older athlete is still greater than we know. We're learning more every day as more older athletes, especially women, are training smarter and performing at higher levels than ever before.

Biographical Doubts

Some doubts women have relate to their history.

Doubt #5: I can't or shouldn't take time from others. A woman at my stage in life isn't supposed to take time from others to focus on a new sport....Many women feel guilty taking time

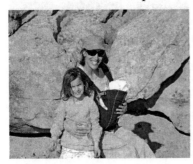

Sarah Keller and her daughters Chloe and Cale on the Rim Rocks in Mountana.

for themselves. Sarah Keller is the mother of two, college professor of communications, and the runner and triathlete you met in Capter 6. Pursuing sports in adulthood has been a central and successful part of her life. But it took years before she didn't feel guilty "going for it". "I grew up in an academic family which felt that sports in adulthood was trivial, that they were something you should outgrow," she said. "But I always had a natural passion for the outdoors so I took up triathlon at 30," she said. "When I got my first job as a professor, I felt as if I should give up triathlon even though I didn't. Triathlon was a source of identity, friends, and happiness and balance. Over the years, I have continued to find ways to combine athletics with professional career and family."

A number of the women masters runners in my dissertation said they felt others frowned on their running pursuits. They said things like: "People think middle-aged women are supposed to sit down somewhere," "You're supposed to fade away into athletic obscurity and into family, taking care of parents or children or career," and "Some people resent it that you're out there on the roads doing something physical and they're not. They wonder why don't you go get in your rocking chair and give up?'"

What these people don't realize is the difference working on and achieving an athletic goal makes in building a better life for yourself and your family, getting you engaged in your career or even helping you change it for the better. Stay away from skeptics. Surround yourself with people who support you and search for role models. If you look, they'll turn up – on the internet, in your neighborhood, in athletic clubs in your area. Many athletic clubs and organizations have divisions not only for women over 30 but also for five-year groups from 30 to 90 and over.

If you don't find a role model, be the pioneer. It's an opportunity….and there are rewards to being the first.

Doubt #6: It's too late to learn something new at my age. Younger people will show me up – that will be embarrassing. Many women say this doubt keeps them from trying something new. It's true. Younger people often learn faster. Jane Morse confirmed this. Remember Jane? She joined her first rowing class at age 55 at Community Rowing in Boston and appropriately took on the beginner's mind. She flipped her rowing scull in the first class. The other beginners in her class were a generation younger: "In my first sculling class it was me and five kids in their 20s. They all picked it up much faster than I did. I fell out of my single. They didn't. I went swimming in the Charles three or four times. It was obvious that the younger people were learning faster."

If you are deterred by that doubt, consider the ten-year rule and Morse's experience. It did take Morse longer to get started than it did younger beginning rowers. But remember as well what she accomplished – winning the Head of the Charles and the Canadian Henley for her age group. Age did not hold her back. But she had the right attitude, persisted, had talent, and got far. No matter when you start, research shows that given equal amounts of talent and hours of practice, it is possible to attain the same levels of achievement as those who started when young.[15]

---

15. Utzschneider, Women Runners.

Doubt #7: I was a strong athlete – I even coached. I can't begin again. I'd like to do something new but it's hard to picture myself starting something all over again....not sure I'm up for that. I may feel stupid. Has-been or former elite athletes often feel as conflicted about taking on a new sport as never-been athletes. Egos based on former prowess deter some from learning something new.

High school and college tennis player Debby Green understands. In her late 30s, she stopped playing tennis due to a foot injury. "If I couldn't play at the level I was used to, I didn't want to play at all. Shutting it off was easier." At 40, she took up cycling. Her husband liked it, and it didn't require the logistical hassles of scheduling court time, finding partners, etc. "There are advantages and disadvantages to having had an athletic history," she said. "The advantage is that you know what it takes to work hard and to accomplish something at a high level.

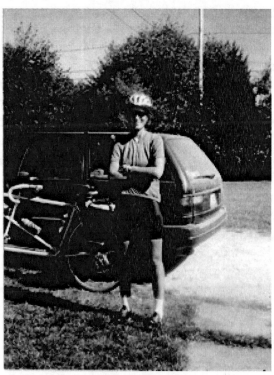

Debby Green ready for a training ride.

"The disadvantage is that you feel weird starting something new. You are not used to feeling powerless, uncoordinated, and not in control. It's awkward, embarrassing and potentially demoralizing. You're used to being the teacher, the one who's looked up to. You'd almost rather not put yourself in that position."

When you have these thoughts, it's time to put yourself back in the "beginner's mind". You do have the right to be a beginner again, to try something new. Chances are you'll live longer than your mother. Why spend years looking back? Also, who cares if you're awkward? No one cares about how you look as much as you do.

Doubt #8. Me? An Athlete? Ridiculous! The thought of me – an athlete -- ridiculous. I am not particularly coordinated and am *NOT* competitive! That's not my self-image. Some women say they remember all too well a moment in sports when they defined themselves as a "forever klutz". "I was in eighth grade playing softball," said one self-proclaimed non-athlete. "I didn't have good hand-eye coordination. So I was nervous when it was my turn to bat," she said. "And then some people on the other team started calling me '1 – 2 – 3!'. The implication was three strikes and I'd be out. I've stayed away from sports since."

Unfortunately, many women say they don't think of themselves as athletes because sports were not encouraged at home or in school. Gynecologist Dr. Nina Carroll never saw herself as an athlete until her late 40s. "I was 48, menopausal, and I didn't exercise regularly," she said. "I was concerned about my bones and wanted to establish a regular exercise habit but had no idea how to begin....I had never really run and was about nine pounds over my ideal weight." Her first time, she ran 10 single minutes with walking breaks between.

"I remember the exact moment I realized I was an athlete," she said. "I was taking off my warm-up clothes before a race and seeing these fabulously fit people in their running clothes...and I thought 'If I'm here with them, then I must be an athlete too!' That was such a startling realization. I was 52, and it changed my whole perception and motivation."

Doubt #9: I don't want to compete. I dislike competing or I'm tired of competing or I'm nervous that a sport might bring out a hidden competitive spirit in me. Then I'll want to be as good as I can be, even the best. Are my friends going to resent me then? These are common complaints.

With regard to the first two, there's no need to compete. An athletic goal doesn't have to involve competition. With regard to the third, there's nothing wrong with being competitive and wanting to be or do your best. Sports can be an opportunity for challenge, spirit, and fun. If putting your heart into something you love means turning off friends, you may want to find others with whom to enjoy sports.

Doubt #10: I have too much going on already – my schedule is way too hectic. You feel like you're dreaming if you think you can add a sport to your already overloaded schedule. You're busy. You've got a job, maybe a spouse or partner, children and carpools, or a family member who needs care. Who has time or energy to focus on a new sport? Just staying in shape is a challenge. For the 103 women runners in my study, too many responsibilities were the major obstacle to success. Too many commitments posed greater obstacles than the slowing effect of aging, injury, or the effects of menopause (which, they say, were minor).

"I feel like I have a double life," said one avid swimmer. "I've got my swimming life and I've got my children and circle of friends. There is a potential conflict with friends. There is the potential problem of turning friends off. I have had to compromise. Of course my family has to come first."

It is true. Too many commitments can be a major obstacle to any achievement. There are years in your life – even clusters of years – when it may not be the right time for an athletic goal. Be careful not to use that as a general excuse, however, denying yourself the benefits of an athletic goal.

If you think you want something new, though, despite – or because of – your commitments, examine your schedule and priorities. Sometimes even in a very busy day, doing something athletic makes the day more tolerable and, often, more efficient. You might be surprised if you really parse your obligations and timetable, that there just may be room for this goal. Say "no" to things that are not a priority. An athletic goal may just end up the most important and enjoyable commitment you have.

Doubt #11. It's too much of a hurdle to just get started. Getting started is hard, say many women who began a new sport. Many have no idea how to go about it. Tennis player Claire Williams talked about the challenges of starting tennis. "Having never focused on any one sport, I had little experience and saw no clear path, no clear way to get on the road to tennis. The hurdles to training seemed larger than the potential rewards. It was confusing, at first. I didn't know where this was going to lead. Either way it went, it could be bad. If it went well, it could develop into a huge commitment and if it went poorly then I had failed. Who wants to be mediocre?"

When you are in high school or college, you have a catalogue of recreational activities from which to choose. They are all reasonably close to you and you are expected to be active. Now, out in the world at whatever age, the options are overwhelming. Should you try karate or yoga or rowing? How do you start something that you're unsure of in the first place? Well, *MOVE!*

More and more communities are creating public programs for adults. Check your local phone book. Talk with others… those who know you, those you may not know well but who are involved in some activity you might be thinking about. That's what Kathleen Mulroy did. She took up rowing at 54. She had been a runner since her twenties and had recently been plagued by meniscus issues. "One of my knees would chronically flare up and I had surgery on my other knee," she said. "I could run three or four miles but didn't want to get to the place where I couldn't run at all." Having heard about rowing from her daughter and neighbor, she tried a novice sweep – rowing in which one holds one oar with both hands. She was a member of a boat with eight rowers. "For a woman who missed out on being on a team, this was the best." She loves the team experience, meeting people from all walks of life, and the fact that she's using new muscles, including upper body muscles. "I'm now working out to improve my abilities as a rower," she said. "I'm hooked."

Overcoming doubts is important and easier than you think. To help you, though, I have included a form for just that purpose.

See the **Overcoming Doubts and Fears** form (page 138). So no more excuses. Get out there. *MOVE!*

Overcoming Fears

Fears come in myriad shapes and sizes. Some people don't take on challenges because of fears, many of which are unfounded. Fears are often buried or masked. A fear of drowning kept Alice Frederick from participating in the triathlon that she had contemplated for four years. A fear of skidding on sand and falling off a bike kept Carol Williamson from participating in a 25 mile bike ride. Doubts about being 15 pounds overweight as well as whether she was athletic enough prevented Melissa from taking on any physical goal. She felt she had to lose the pounds first. She put off trying to find a cycling coach for three years until she realized her doubts were unfounded. She started lifting weights, fast walking, and playing golf, and within a year and a half lost those 15 pounds.

The Overcoming Doubts and Fears form can help you manage fears by asking you to name a major fear and then list as many strategies as possible to overcome it. "Fear of drowning and not being able to swim fast or long enough – I can't swim freestyle for a half mile" was the major fear Alice identified as she contemplated training for a triathlon. She listed 10 techniques to tackle her fear. They included knowing that she could tread water or float on her back anytime, that boats on the course could rescue her, and that she could swim with the slowest swimmers.

"Focusing on and also analyzing the fear help you minimize it," said Alice. "By the time you get to your event, you've anticipated your fear so much that you're almost bored with it. I never panicked during the triathlon and I am looking forward to doing it again next year."

Carol started by biking four days a week for 20 to 25 minutes at a time on an indoor bike. "I was afraid of going downhill so fast I would fall off and hit my head or hit a car. It took me a while to admit that fear. It seemed so silly. Once I was honest about it, I could identify techniques to overcome it," she said.

She joined a bike club, practiced biking in a department store parking lot and switching gears, and bought a rearview mirror for her bike as well as several books on cycling.

"Micromanaging the fear helped shrink it," she said. "Breaking it into bite-size chunks helped so much..... I felt so comfortable after just a month of riding outside that my earlier fear seemed ridiculous. It had kept me from riding for decades so identifying it and addressing it head-on was freeing.

"Learning to brake helped most. You may laugh at this story. It makes me look like the ultimate nerd. But hey, it worked......On one of the first days I went out with a triathlon coach for advice on braking. Like many beginners, I had made the mistake of braking the whole way down hills. If you do that, you wear out the brake pads. The coach told me to practice braking in spurts instead. After riding down a long hill, I asked if we could stop for a minute or two because I wanted to write that tip down. I was afraid I would forget it. We've been laughing about that ever since. I am still riding distance events. I'm not interested in riding fast, but I can bike anywhere and I'm not afraid of hills."

Melissa, who felt she had to lose the 15 pounds before taking on a goal, talked about her changed attitude: "How many women say they're not going to do something – buy a bathing suit, a dress, whatever – until they lose weight? I finally acknowledged that my extra weight was an excuse." Melissa overcame her doubts about waiting to start any athletic endeavor until after she lost weight. The Franklin Roosevelt quote, "The only thing to fear is fear itself," is one of her favorites. "I went for it," she said. "I started training and – it took a number of months (five or six) – but most of the weight came off."

Overcoming Doubts and Fears -- Completed

Given your goal, what is a major hurdle or fear that could harm your enjoyment and performance? (If you face hurdles, you may complete this form several times.)

1. <u>I am petrified to bike outside – afraid of going too fast downhill, that I will fall and hit a car or hit my head.</u>

> Can you identify a technique – mental, physical, or logistical – that will help you deal with the hurdle?

1. <u>Look into bike clubs for a beginner group to learn how to train for distance biking. A coach there can give me advice about what kind of bike and helmet to buy.</u>

2. <u>I will start by only biking with a group, and I will avoid hills until I learn how to use the brakes and gears.</u>

3. <u>I need to buy a helmet, water bottle, pump, and repair kit – the biking coach can help with that.</u>

4. <u>Remember that I don't have to do everything at once. I am going to take this step by step.</u>

5. <u>Get padded, comfortable seat helps balance on a bike. I'll get one.</u>

6. <u>Don't feel I have to buy those shoes that lock into the pedals. I am taking this one step at a time.</u>

"No matter how far life pushes you down, no matter how much you hurt, you can always bounce back." -Sheryl Swoopes

Overcoming Doubts and Fears -- Completed

7. Don't compare yourself to anyone else...... If I find this out-door cycling thing isn't for me, "sayonara"! I'll try something else.

8. Figure out whether my glasses will work with outdoor biking.... Maybe get something that will keep them on?

9. Buy Cycling Past 50 by Joe Friel.

Statement that you will overcome that doubt or fear:

I WILL OVERCOME MY FEAR OF FALLING AND COMFORT IN A PACK!

I WILL OVERCOME MY DOUBTS ABOUT MY KNEE ACTING UP.

"No matter how far life pushes you down, no matter how much you hurt, you can always bounce back." -Sheryl Swoopes

Managing Goals: Setbacks

"The world is full of suffering but
it is also full of people overcoming it."
- Helen Keller

---

*A setback is any reversal -- personal, physical, or professional –
that disrupts your progress.*

*To avoid injury, listen to your body! Moderation, rest, cross
training, stretching and strengthening, and a healthy diet helps
ward off injury.*

*Once injured, be your own best advocate in terms of seeking
professional advice. Get a second or third opinion.*

*Remember: setbacks don't mean failure. Be flexible and patient.
Extend the time to achieve your goal.*

Great – you overcame your doubts and fears, you set your goals, and you felt good as soon as you wrote them down. Then the starting gun goes off, you take your first few strides... and life unfolds. "Stuff" starts happening. Real life gets in the way of your training. You're caught off guard, you start feeling discouraged, frustrated, perhaps hopeless. The paper with your goals on it ends up in the trash, along with the realization that setting goals was either just a fun or unproductive activity one afternoon a few weeks ago. You let go of that dream (it was just a whim, anyway). Like a balloon, it drifts up and off into blue skies. *Au revoir!* See you again? Maybe someday, you say.

For ultimate success, it is so important to remember: *the road to achieving long-term goals is never smooth*. There are *always* setbacks, and discouraging events that block your path. Always. And everyone has them. It's hard to anticipate some setbacks and difficult to avoid being discouraged. This chapter discusses both physical and other setbacks, including professional and personal setbacks, and what you can do, if anything, to prevent some of them and how you can deal with the rest of them.

Setbacks

A setback here is defined as anything that significantly disrupts your training – anything that throws you off for more than a week. Setbacks come in all shapes and sizes and generally fall into one of three categories: physical, professional, or personal. Note that good things – like promotions and moving or buying a new house – can be setbacks in your training. They can be positive setbacks but they are setbacks, nonetheless. Setbacks may be the result of something that happens to you or to someone close to you. If you're sick, that's a setback. If your child or parent is sick, that's a setback. If you lose your job, you're thrown off course. If your spouse loses a job, your life balance is also upset. In <u>Overwhelmed: Coping With Life's Ups and Downs</u>, Nancy Schlossberg emphasizes that any change in your life or in another's life will affect the roles, relationships, and routines of others around you.[16]

Simply put, life is fraught with change, and change will affect your training. You may not encounter a setback on the way to your first short-term goal, but sooner or later you're bound to meet one. What should you do? Scale back your training temporarily (but only if you have to). Extend the time to achieve your goal. When you return to training, return at a level reduced from where it was (the degree to which you return depends on your circumstances). **Whatever you do, don't let go of your goals completely.** As Winston Churchill once said, "never, never, never give up."

Physical Setbacks. Physical setbacks are injuries (first-time injuries and "hello-don't forget me - I'm-here-again" injuries), sickness, disease or just fatigue. You may pull a muscle. Get the flu. You may even get sick – really sick, God forbid. Some women with cancer, however, have trained for all kinds of goals, albeit at a reduced degree. In my study of over 100 masters runners, 80 percent said that they had experienced injuries that kept them from running for an average of three and one-half months. Most common among these were stress fractures, hamstring strains, and groin pulls. And though the average age of these women was 52, fewer than 15% said that menopause had affected them negatively.[17]

You Can Ward Off Injury. You can take precautions to avoid injury. I have a "Stay Healthy Checklist" which I give to clients that includes the following:

> • *Be moderate in your approach.* Don't obsess and lose perspective. Moderation was one quality that the masters women runners in my study said made them successful. "You must start out and not be the best right away,"

---

16. Nancy Schlossberg, Overwhelmed: Coping With Life's Ups and Downs (New York: M. Evans & Company, 2007).

17. Utzschneider, Women Runners.

said another woman, "You can't let running or anything be an obsession. You'll burn out. Don't over train and let your sport run your life. Obsession takes the fun out of sports."

• *Respect the importance of rest.* Rest recharges you. If you gradually increase your training over three weeks, incorporate a lighter, "cut-back" week during the fourth week to recharge your body. "If I'm hurting I don't run," said a runner. "I'll take a couple of days off. I just had a virus and took six days off. It gives your body a chance to recover. The older you get, the smarter you have to be."

• *Cross train.* Exercise differently from your usual routine (swimming instead of playing tennis, biking instead of running) if your body feels tired or you begin to feel an injury coming on. Cross training will prevent you from obsessing and losing perspective. If you feel a soreness in the same spot for three days in a row, cross train for at least three days to see if the soreness goes away. Make the switch immediately to prevent injury. Say you pull your rotator cuff and are a swimmer. Switch to biking right away – or run. Runners with various injuries that prevent running can run in the water or use the elliptical machine or the bike. I've trained Olympic marathon trials runners in the water after they were diagnosed with stress fractures. They ran in the water for three months and were only on land for the month before the marathon. They did as well as their competitors who had been on land the entire time. With most kinds of cross training (depending on your sport), you won't be using the same muscles you need for your main sport. But it's good to keep your muscles moving and your blood flowing. The sooner you change your exercise after feeling a pain, the better. A rule of thumb – if you feel discomfort for more than three days in a row of the same activity, *stop that activity!* Consult your coach about the best alternative exercises.

• *Listen to your body.* It sounds obvious, but more often than not, women report painful areas months after they've felt discomfort in one place. Acknowledge soreness as soon as you feel it and if you feel it three days in a row, take a few days off before testing the activity again. If you continue to feel pain, stop immediately and cross train.

• *If you're over 30, be sure to incorporate strength training and stretching* into your routine, even if that totals 30 minutes three times a week. It's worth it. We lose a half a pound of muscle each year after 30 without strength training. We lose elasticity in our joints. Yoga is an alternative that combines both stretching and strengthening. You don't necessarily need a gym with machines. You can do exercises that use your own body weight. Basic strength training exercises are push-ups, sit-ups, and sitting leg lifts, for example.

• *Eat a healthy diet* with plenty of fruit, vegetables and dairy products. Adequate hydration – drinking at least eight 8 ounce glasses of water daily and more depending on how much you exercise – helps maintain normal joint function (cartilage is 65 to 80% water) and prevents dehydration in general. Check with your doctor that you consume enough calcium, protein, and iron. Vitamin D, for example, is required for calcium absorption. The best source of vitamin D is sunshine for approximately 20 minutes per day. A general recommendation is to take at least a daily multi-vitamin and also 1200 milligrams of fish or flaxseed oil.

• *Research alternative healing techniques* including acupuncture or active release therapy (a movement based massage technique that treats problems with muscles, tendons, ligaments, fascia, and nerves) which some people find helpful. You could also try trigger point therapy, a touch therapy practiced by a broad range of healthcare providers including chiropractors, medical doctors, physical therapists, and massage therapists. Trigger points are tender or painful areas of the body which, when pressed deeply enough, stimulate the nervous system and increase circulation to promote healing.

• *Consult with your coach or more experienced friend* about treating yourself. Learn a tip about sitting or lying on a roller or tennis ball to massage a sore area of your body.

<u>Whoops! You're Injured.</u> What can you do about an injury once you have one? The first thing for many sports injuries and the best form of first aid that you can control is easy to remember. Think R-I-C-E, Rest, Ice, Compression, and Elevation. This practice is helpful for a wide range of injuries from sprains, strains, simple fractures, and dislocations. As soon as you realize you have an injury, rest. You don't want to aggravate it. Why ice? You may have internal bleeding from injured blood vessels. Ice causes small blood vessels to contract. That decreases the amount of blood that can collect around the wound and thereby speeds healing. The more blood that collects around the wound, the longer the healing time. Compression means you wrap the injured or sore area with an elastic bandage. Don't wrap it too tightly, since this can cause more swelling below the affected area. Wrapping decreases swelling, slows bleeding and keeps blood from healthy tissue from entering the injured site and accumulating. Elevation of the injured area – raising it above the level of your heart — can also help limit swelling and pain.

As soon as possible, both check with your doctor and talk with as many people as you can, including your coach and more experienced friends about various specialists. There are more sports medicine specialists than ever, and each one has a different approach to the same injury. A chiropractor, physical therapist, physiatrist (a medical doctor and nerve, muscle, and bone expert who treats injuries or illnesses that affect how you move), an orthopedist (a doctor who also specializes in spine and the musculoskeletal system), acupuncturist, and a neurosurgeon are all going to treat a neck pain differently.

To complicate matters further, each specialist varies within each discipline. Talking to as many people as you can will help you find the best practitioner for you. Listen to your doctor, but also get a second opinion. *Most of all, listen to your body.* Many times a second opinion contradicts a first opinion. Sometimes even the most hallowed doctors are wrong. I was told by one orthopedic surgeon that I could not run more than two miles a week in my mid-forties. Since then I have been running more than 30 miles a week for the past ten years with no problems. I have been told by a chiropractor that my hamstring would take 40 weeks to heal. I was back running after five weeks. In each case, though, I was careful in how I approached my injury, taking care not to push through any pain whatsoever.

When dealing with an injury, remember that people have different tolerances for pain as well as different time requirements for healing. While in a sport you may be in competition with others, when it comes to healing you are not competing with anyone else. Again, listen to your doctor and listen to your own body. It's good to be inspired by others but their bodies are different. You have to follow your own body. There is no need to feel guilty or discouraged if your healing process is slower than others. It is just important to *heal in your own time at your own pace.*

Inform yourself to the greatest degree possible about all resources for your injury. Read about it – on-line, at the library, or in the bookstore. Books that may help you understand your injury are The Complete Guide to Sports Injuries by H. Winter Griffith (Penguin Group, 2004) and an older, excellent book, the Sports Injury Handbook: Professional Advice for Amateur Athletes by Allan Levy and Mark Fuerst (1993, John Wiley & Sons, Inc.). Talk with friends who may have also have experienced your injury and, most important, consult with several doctors including some who may have different perspectives on it. As mentioned earlier, innovative therapies are available which help the body repair, replace, restore, and regenerate damaged or diseased musculoskeletal tissue. Some of these therapies are non-surgical and minimally invasive.

If you have a chronic injury that has not responded to six months of traditional treatment, you might want to interview doctors at hospitals and centers familiar with these treatments. For instance, in Boston, where I am, a leading institution of new regenerative non-surgical treatment is the Spaulding Rehabilitation Center in Wellesley, MA. Knowing that these treatments exist will help you decide whether they are something to consider. *I am not recommending any particular therapy here but, again, getting medical advice for any therapy from several doctors, is essential.*

Take time to build your cardiovascular endurance. Even though you are injured, you can usually stay in great shape through cross training and building up your cardiovascular endurance, the most important aspect of fitness. Cardiovascular endurance is the ability of the heart, blood, blood vessels, and respiratory system to provide oxygen and fuel to muscles to perform a particular exercise for a considerable amount of time at a steady rate. You can build cardiovascular endurance with running, biking, a step machine, rowing, swimming, water running, jumping rope, and with continuous exercises such as sit-ups, push-ups, chin-ups, etc. If you're injured, you can usually find one kind of exercise you're able to continue. If you're injured from swimming or rowing, for example, you may be able to bike or run, etc. If possible, begin with 20 minutes of exercise. If 20 minutes are too much, exercise for a few minutes at a time and intersperse a minute of rest between efforts so the exercises total 20 minutes by the end of the workout. You can build from there. Endurance training can change muscle tissue increasing mitochondrial and capillary density, metabolic enzyme activity, and glycogen storage. The good news: this means greater performance when you return to your sport of choice. But remember to avoid re-injury. When you return to your normal activity, return at a much reduced level and, again, consult with a physician for advice.

Like most of us, elite masters runner Coreen Steinbach has learned how to handle injuries from experience. Before her first injury, she dismissed a persistent twinge. "If I had a workout planned I pretty much did it come hell or high water," she said. One year, a pain that she was trying to push through became chronic. "I accepted it as the status quo… That fall I had a pain in my butt that would come and go, lessen and intensify, but always be there," she said. "The problem became one I could not ignore." She ordered an MRI, which showed a severe tear of the hamstring with an avulsion from the bone – an area where the ligaments and tendons had torn from the bone.

"It was not good," she said. She stopped running for seven

weeks and became a "rehab beast." She immediately ruled out surgery and studied everything there was to know about her injury.

She consulted a number of experts including a physical therapist and an orthopedic surgeon. "Ultimately, I crafted a rehabilitation program myself," she said. "I quickly learned that no one person could tell me what to do…. I formulated an action plan to address the weaknesses that led to this injury in the first place and implemented a regime to strengthen the weak side." Her rehabilitation program (a little more intense than the average person's) included:

- acupuncture twice a week for the first month
- Active Release Therapy (ART), soft tissue movement-based massage, and physical therapy including deep tissue massage once a week
- "lots" of cross training including 90 minutes of pool running every third day and training on the elliptical and other machines
- light weight training to strengthen her legs from the dorsiflexors to the hips and
- core (lower back and abdominal muscles) and balance work.

That's not all.

"I improved my nutrition," she said. A vegetarian for 27 years, she focused on increasing protein intake to help heal her injury. She began taking whey powder and increased intake of zinc to aid the healing process. She also cut down on coffee as its acidity detracted from healing. "This was how my husband knew I was serious," she said.

When she started running again, she took it "slowly, ever so slowly. I started walking 5 minutes and then running 5," she said. Exactly a year after she stopped racing she was back on the track for a race. "It is not hyperbole to say that I cried tears of joy."

"The most important lesson I learned is that you MUST be your own advocate when it comes to rehabilitation. You have to take it upon yourself to craft a program that will return you to running. There just doesn't seem to be a consensus among physicians, physical therapists, coaches, etc. as to what works or sometimes what the injury even is!!"

After getting advice from more than one source and experts, remember that you are ultimately responsible for your own healing. Most importantly, listen to your body and don't rush the healing process. Instead work around (but don't aggravate) your injury. You'll be more fit and stronger when you return to your sport.

Professional And Personal Setbacks

Personal and professional setbacks is a catch-all category for the thousands of events which throw us off course. They are too numerous and idiosyncratic to list. They're life. Your child gets sick. You get sick. You lose your job, or your husband loses his. You adopt a child. You move. You get promoted and feel excited but overwhelmed. A family member or friend dies. Usually, but not always, setbacks take us by surprise.

How do you handle setbacks? There are thousands of answers. My suggestion is to maintain as much of your training as possible. It helps you maintain a sense of balance when all else around you is in chaos.

Leni Webber maintained her training through a number of setbacks including a layoff, dealing with a struggling adolescent, moving her ailing, octogenarian mother from California to Massachusetts, and dealing with grief over her mother's eventual death.

"When you feel things are out of control, you've got to try to get as much control as you can," she said. "I saw no reason to abandon the consistency and predictability and sense of pleasure my training gave me during some of the most difficult times of my life." Did she ever feel guilty training during these times, that she should have been doing something else? "No," she answered promptly. "The only challenging part was making sure to fit it in and I found I needed to work a little harder to fit it in but it was never a question of dropping it out."

How would she have felt if she had dropped training and tended to the setbacks? "I would have felt that I was letting the setbacks take over and that I wasn't being fair to myself because, if anything, I needed more strength than ever."

Do Setbacks Lead To Failure?

Yes and no. If you think that you can accomplish your goal only in a particular time period, then yes, setbacks lead to failure. If you're willing to take more time to achieve your goal, then the answer is no. Take more time to achieve your goal.

One of the key tenets of MOVE! and one which cannot be emphasized enough – is that, as long as you are willing to continue striving towards your goal and modify it, if necessary, to meet your interests and circumstances, you do not fail. You will eventually achieve your goal.

Assessing Goals and Achievements

"Everyone thinks of changing the world,
but no one thinks of changing himself."
- Leo Tolstoy

Assessing goals and achievements is invaluable.

It helps you evaluate what worked and what didn't.

Objective assessments help you refine future goals.

You gain perspective on your achievements by noting challenges overcome and surprise accomplishments you hadn't planned for when they happened.

MOVE!

Why bother looking back once you've achieved your goal? Why look back if you didn't achieve it? If you're like most people you just want to move on. After all, analysis and reflection are time consuming. Looking to the past is not particularly helpful because now you, your body, and your circumstances have changed. Right?

Wrong. Your athletic history as recorded in your training journal is a goldmine of information – information that is invaluable for achieving your current goal and setting your next one. It is there that you have unique information about yourself. It is there you can get a clear picture of what distractions you tend to encounter – are they avoidable or unavoidable, what workouts you are able to handle easily, which ones are difficult, which lead to injury, rest days which helped your performance, etc. Taking a half hour to review what took several months to accomplish can teach you the keys to your athletic success.

I can't stress enough how important it is to review and assess where you are and where you've been as you work to achieve your various goals.

Make It A Habit: Review Your Goals

Make it a habit to review your short-term goals once a week and your annual goal once a month. You'll remind yourself of your priorities. The forms either will confirm the path you're on or suggest goals that need to be revised. You are more likely to want to revise your annual rather than your short-term goal. Are annual athletic goals and annual goals in other areas of life still relevant, still possible? If not, revise them – and note the dates on which you wrote the changes. Remember: goals have to be flexible.

"I like looking over my long-term goals for a number of reasons," said swimmer Martha Gibson. "I have a lot going on so I often forget what my main goals are, both athletic and non-athletic. Also, sometimes I change them. This year one of my main goals was to reorganize our basement. Then my mother

154

got sick and I changed my focus to include helping her. I gave up the basement goal. Some of life isn't planned, and obviously I couldn't have predicted my mother's situation."

Post-Goal Analysis

Post-goal analysis, once goals are achieved or not achieved, is essential. Forms most helpful for this exercise of looking back are

- the Short-Term Goal Review,
- the Post-Goal Analysis and
- the Annual Goal Review.

The Short-Term Goal Review. The **Short-Term Goal Review** (page 156) gives you a chance to evaluate, post-goal, how realistic or challenging your short-term goal was. The form asks you to rate how well you trained for successful completion of a general goal. Referring back to your Short-Term Goal Review, you can see what your specific training goals were and then note how you would rate your training on a scale of 1 to 5. The form also asks you to note challenges overcome and also what you learned in the process of training.

It's a quick form to fill out and it will help you set your next short-term goal. If, for example, you set a goal that included doing 25 to 30 push-ups three to four times a week and you only did ten twice a week, you will know that your next short-term goal should have a more moderate goal for push-ups or that you should choose another upper body strength training method – or that you should leave it out altogether, depending on your next goal.

The Post-Goal Analysis. The **Post-Goal Analysis** (page 158) asks you to summarize your process or preparation for your particular goal. The form is general on purpose. You can tailor it to your needs. One person's training looks entirely different from another's. Hiker Cheryl Suchors used the form multiple

Short-Term Goal Review -- Completed

Beginning Date: _July 1, 2011_
Ending Date: _August 12, 2011_

Did you reach your goal? Yes __X__   No _____

Rate your performance on the following applicable components on a scale of 1 to 5, with 1 representing weakest and 5 representing greatest effort:

Cardiovascular training: ____5____
Intensity: ____3____
Strength: ____4____
Flexibility: ____4____
Mental (reading, meditations, vision statements, etc.): ____3____
Skill development: ____3____
Nutrition: ____4____
Other (balance, coordination): ____3____

Challenges overcome:

1. _Maintained training schedule during trip to Maine._

2. _Planned my schedule well. Ran early or late during heat wave._

3. _Cross trained during the week my hamstrings felt sore._

4. _____

5. _____

"Champions keep playing until they get it right." -Billie King

Short-Term Goal Review -- Completed

What have you learned in this process?

1. _I am able to stick to a reasonable goal (45 minutes_

a day for training) even on a family vacation.

2. _____

Are other commitments being met?

Re: reorganization of basement. I am two-thirds done. Still
need to organize the bookshelves. Slightly disappointed but
Katie was sick. Can juggle other non-athletic commitments
to finish it.

"Champions keep playing until they get it right." -Billie King

Post-Goal Analysis -- Completed

Event: _5K Freihofer's June 2010_

1. What was your event goal? _To run under 19:10_

2. What was you actual result? _19:02_

3. What were your hopes? _I wanted to break 19:10._

4. What were your fears? _I wouldn't stay focused in the third quarter of the race._

5. On a scale of 1 to 10 with 10 representing "Most" and "1" representing "Least", how would you rate your....

      Physical readiness -- _9_

      Mental readiness -- _8_

6. Comments on any particular circumstances to note related to the day of the event (logistics, weather, etc.)?

This was a terrific day. Proved that I can achieve my goals with patience and consistency. It was cooler than when I ran it last year. I was alone (last time went with another runner, but now concluding that this is not ideal for me). Arrived 1 hour before race, which helped me de-stress about logistics and focus. Weather good — 62 degrees.

Post-Goal Analysis -- Completed

7. Summarize your weekly physical and mental training over the past 3 months (duration, intensity, frequency of workouts – drills, etc.)

Physical Training and Mental Training (Review of Weekly Training Journal):

Weekly routine, 3 months (weeks 8 – 12) before the event:

38 – 44 miles per week, one tempo run (25 to 30 minutes) and one interval workout (2.5 – 3.0 miles of intervals). One long run of 10 – 12 miles per week. Drills three times a week. Weight training twice per week. Dynamic stretching 5X week.

Mental training -- just wrote down training in journal

Weekly routine, 2 months (weeks 4 – 7) before the event:

40– 45 miles per week, one tempo run (30 to 35 minutes) and one interval workout (2.5 – 3.0 miles of intervals) per week. Weekly long run 9 – 11 miles, same drills and weights. Two "training" races (Fresh Pond races). Two hill workouts. Kept on with drills, weights, and stretching.

Mental training -- did a few affirmations before threshold workouts ("I feel strong when I run long"). Need to improve.

Weekly routine, 1 month (weeks 0 – 4) before the event:

40 to 42 miles per week. one tempo run (30 to 40 minutes) and one interval workout (2.5 – 3.0 miles of intervals) per week except for the last week. Weekly long run 9 – 11 miles, drills and weights. One "training" race (Fresh Pond). Two hill workouts. Kept drill, weights, stretch routine.

During the last two weeks visualized race course and segmented distance with "cue" works – "easy and relaxed" for first 1.5 miles, "steady and strong" for next mile, and "quick and smooth: for last .6 miles.

"When I go out on the ice, I just think about my skating. I forget it is a competition."
-Katarina Witt

159

Post-Goal Analysis -- Completed

8. What other life events (related to work, personal life, events of the day etc.) affected – helped or hindered – your training over the past 3 months?

This was a good stretch of training. One week during the second month was tough. Marc got the flu , I had volunteered to do an extra marketing project for the office, and I hosted our book group. Too much.

9. If you attempt that same or another goal, how would you improve your training?

Be better at saying "no". When I'm planning a race, look ahead and see what else is going on. I didn't have to host the book group at the same time that the extra project was due. Am I crazy?! Realize that I am not superwoman. Respect a few commitments. Next time plan the book group at another time . Should have been realistic about how much work the marketing project involves.

Other Comments:

In June I was a little distracted by the arrival and training of a new puppy, and by several sets of house guests. Otherwise this was a terrific experience and I can't believe I achieved this goal because I am faster now than I was five years ago! These races make me feel stronger as I get older, and the clock is proof of that. I actually looking forward to moving up to a new age category.

"When I go out on the ice, I just think about my skating. I forget it is a competition."
-Katarina Witt

times, having achieved her goal in a ten-year span of "bagging" the 48 4,000-Footers in New Hampshire. Her training for Mount Madison, for example, included yoga, stretch training, knee exercises, elliptical training and Nordic track workouts, massage, icing, visualizations, acupuncture and more. For runner Antonia Hieronymous, on the other hand, preparing to run a five kilometer race, her training involved stretching, drills, visualizations, strength training, occasional cross training, drinking at least 64 ounces of water daily, and running at easy, moderately intense, and intense paces.

The Post-Goal Analysis is a powerful tool for evaluating your training for a major event. It asks you to summarize your weekly physical and mental training over the three months prior to the event and to recall what other life events have helped or hindered you. The form also asks how you might improve your training were you to do the same or a similar event again.

It asks about:

- your goal and your actual result,
- the number of weeks of training involved,
- whether or not you had any specific physical weaknesses or injuries at the beginning of or during any of the training,
- how ready you were physically and mentally on the day of the event (on a scale of one to ten),
- any circumstances related to logistics, and weather conditions during the event that would be helpful to remember, and
- any thoughts you have about the experience in general.

Many of my athletes keep this form for years as a useful reference for creating future goals and future events. The Post-Goal Analysis helps you …

…remember the details of your training.

Most people have a hard time remembering details from three days ago. "I'm likely to have forgotten tons of things, both good and bad, that were important in the process," said Cheryl.

"For me, I always have other than physical training goals. I am a person who works hard at things, but I forget how hard I've worked. I forget how much the day by day, step by step, hour by hour adds up to achieving goals. Life is always more than one thing. While I was trying to hike my mountains I was also parenting my daughter, changing careers, and trying to be a good wife and activist. Writing down your achievements is a way of keeping your eye on the most important things. It's a way of not getting deflected or unfocused."

... remember the goal objectively.

After completing a goal or an event, we can feel so emotional that we don't remember what led to it. If we didn't perform as well as we had hoped we don't want to think about it. If we did very well, we are generally ebullient. Our feelings distort the facts.

"Sometimes you get so excited that you accomplished something that you can't remember why you did well," said tennis player Lisa Steinberg. "Until I completed the Post-Goal Analysis, I didn't realize that one reason I achieved my goal of raising my tennis rating was that I practiced my volleys and overheads at least twice a week. I had forgotten that completely."

...get perspective.

"The Post-Goal Analysis puts the goal or event in the perspective of something that comes at the end of a process, " said Lisa. "There has been this whole process that you've engaged in. Half the time I forget what happened when I was getting ready for my event....I forget that I got sick or that my son was sick or that I had to go to California to see my mother in the middle of training. As amazing as it sounds, it makes me feel good about myself and my achievement."

...celebrate if you reached your goal.

Without it, there is often a feeling of letdown and a lack of perspective. "The Post-Goal Analysis is wonderful because it's immediate," Cheryl added. "It's a way of celebrating the victory.

There are very few people you can talk with about your physical victory who will understand it or understand what it means to you and all that you've been through to make it happen. It's a way of debriefing that allows you to live through it again. If it was a victory that's delicious! If it wasn't a victory it's a place to vent your disappointment and in a way that lets you feel you can take some control over what didn't work and why. It puts you back in charge."

...see why you didn't reach your goal.

Martha Gibson set a goal of swimming a half mile in 20 minutes, which she didn't achieve. She swam it in 22 minutes. Completing the Post-Goal Analysis she realized the goal was too aggressive. She started from a baseline of being able to swim six consecutive minutes slowly and she ended up getting a flu for two of the eight weeks. "Next time, I'm going to allow a few weeks for a setback situation," she said.

...improve and refine your process for the future, should you try a similar goal or event.

"What you take away from the particular event that day is nice, but if you don't write things down you will forget a lot," said runner Leni Webber. "It's important data that you have in one place and it is helpful for the future. I can see what I've done well and where I need to tweak my training for a better result. I keep every Post-Goal Analysis, and I do like to look at them. It's like reading a diary or seeing a picture that brings it all back."

After reviewing specific data from previous post-goal analyses, Antonia realized that she could be still faster if she spent more time on moderately intense running – running at 80% of her maximum heart rate twice, rather than once, a week.

"If the event went well, you know you can use that strategy next time," said Antonia. "If it went badly it's good to know those details too. You build up a log. Information is power. The more you know about what works for your training and what doesn't – the more refined you can be. It's all a process of refinement. The goal of training is to make it more and more specific to you. So the more information you have, the better."

...gain insights into yourself above and beyond the athletic achievement, including your ability to commit to and stay focused on future challenges.

Antonia commented in her Post-Goal Analysis that she gained more than achieving her goal. "I smashed my goal and the smile has not left my face," she wrote. "Obviously, in the context of my athletics it is a huge success, but the impact of this race will reach deeply into all aspects of my life. To have the knowledge that I can rise to meet a difficult challenge gives me a confidence about challenges at work and elsewhere. It takes courage to stick your neck out - it may, after all, get chopped off - but life is only the richer for it, even if you fail. I can take total ownership of this achievement. It's mine, and will be forever.

"As I reflect on my race, one thing becomes crystal clear, and that is that training is a process which athletes work at for years and years. Despite disruption in the weeks before the race, I was able to achieve my goal, not because of some miracle but because of the work I've put in over the last three years. Looking forward, I can't choose a future race and decide that that is the day on which I'll peak. It doesn't work like that because injury, work, family, life etc. are unpredictable - but I do know that there are more spectacular races in me that I will run."

The Annual Goal Review. Why bother with an **Annual Goal Review** (page 165) at the end of the year? First, it's helpful to see how you balanced your athletic with other main accomplishments during the year. The form on both athletic and other achievements asks you for a summary of your main physical achievements, surprise milestones, challenges overcome, and achievements in other areas of life. This helps you see all you have juggled in a year. How you complete the forms depends on you and what you consider important.

"The achievements for the year show how far you've come and what you've done," said Antonia. "Human nature is to think about what you haven't done rather than what you have. I think people tend to underestimate their achievements. It's good to step

ASSESSING GOALS AND ACHIEVEMENTS

Annual Goal Review -- Completed

Beginning Date: _August 10th, 2011_
Ending Date: _August 10th, 2012_

1. _Ran the Mount Washington Race – June 18th, 2012._
YES!

2. _Completed the Sturbridge to Bourne Ride (111 miles of_
the Pan Mass Challenge).

SURPRISE MILESTONES

1. _Became comfortable riding with clipless pedals after two_
months of training outdoors!

OTHER COMMITMENTS

1. _Work –Successfully increased consulting business by 15%_
this year.

2. _Decided on assisted living facilities for Mom – finished by_
December as planned.

3. _Established homework routine for kids and they kept to_
it. SUCCESS!

4. _Did NOT join book club! Next year. Wouldn't have had_
time to read everything anyway.

"Hard work has made it easy. That is my secret. That is why I win." -Nadia Comaneci

back and realize how many things you've done, and to see them in one place, to realize 'gosh! I really have done a lot!' Otherwise you don't remember. It helps you put the year in perspective."

What is the point here? Don't sell yourself short. Write down what you've done, what you've achieved. You'll be surprised and walk away with a different attitude.

Surprise Milestones

What is a surprise milestone? It is any accomplishment that you hadn't planned for when it happened.

Surprise milestones for Cheryl related to her writing, training, and personal life. Her entry for surprise milestone #1 was this: "Made first proposal to commercial magazine for first personal essay, first article on hiking. Accepted same day! To be published in Her Sports January/February issue. First photos published, first pay from writing!" Surprise milestone #2 for Cheryl was "Created a chapter-a-month (during non-hiking season) plan; first solid momentum to finish first draft of book." Another surprise milestone was that she completed 70 consecutive minutes on the Nordic Track. "My longest ever!" she wrote.

On her 2007 Annual Review Form, Dr. Barbara Stewart noted not only her main athletic achievement – finishing fourth in her age group in a series of six New England Grand Prix races – but also a surprise milestone of completing a conversion of paper to an electronic medical records system in her practice four months earlier than she had expected. "The discipline of setting weekly training goals seeps into work habits," she said. "The project was completed earlier than expected because of that simple word, discipline. My routine involves setting weekly professional as well as athletic goals." Barbara also noted challenges to master for the next year, including getting to the office by 6:00 a.m. and leaving by 6:00 p.m. "That would help with my life balance," she said. With a handful of exceptions, she did meet that challenge.

Challenges overcome for Barbara included long work hours and a sick step-father; for Antonia, a persistent calf injury; for Karen, a stressful work environment with layoffs; for Leni, multiple trips between California and Massachusetts to care for her aging mother; and, for Cheryl, recovering from chemotherapy.

Other achievements despite the challenges for Barbara, Antonia, Karen, Leni, and Cheryl have varied a great deal from year to year. For Antonia, a photographer, one year they included completing a quilt for her daughter and a photo album she had worked on for years. In addition to installing an electronic medical records system, other achievements for Barbara included completing a professional article. Karen cited finding a better school for her son as one of her other achievements. During one year Leni, an insurance broker, wrote that she increased her client base by 15%. One year, Cheryl mentioned with her other achievements those of her 16-year-old daughter, who had "glowing reports" at school and who had learned how to drive.

Having completed the Annual Goal Review, you'll have learned a lot about your strengths and weaknesses in setting and managing all your goals. You'll know what worked and what didn't. You may even find some surprise accomplishments – those you were not even aware of. Maybe you are motivated to take your goals one step further or maybe you want to stop after you're done. Perhaps you want to try something else altogether. In any event, the Annual Goal Review is a valuable guide to your history of the past year and your potential for the future.

10

Setting The Next Goal

"People always fear change."
- Bill Gates

You may want to continue with another short-term goal or your interests or circumstances may change. You may want to set a goal in a new sport.

- Letting go of an old sport is not easy.
- Keeping a journal, meditating on other possibilities, or talking with friends can help.
- If you want to continue with your sport but at another level, reframe your perspective.
- Is coaching your old sport a possibility?

Having achieved your goal or fallen short, you are either happy with what you accomplished or not. Regardless, you now have two choices. One is to pick another goal in your same sport – either more or less challenging. This can be done easily by reviewing your journal and assessing the process. And remember: *in achieving your goal or in falling short, you achieved something, so give yourself credit.*

Setting the next goal in the same sport simply means returning to the core of the *MOVE!* method which is short-term goal setting. Having many short-term goals and revising them when necessary lead to achieving your long-term goals. Staying with the same sport is effective because you gather so much information about what works for you and what doesn't.

But if you didn't enjoy the sport, don't be hesitant to change sports, whether it's a new sport you became intrigued with a few months ago or one you've done forever. Sometimes switching is simple. Sometimes it isn't – particularly when you've been very involved in a sport over much of your life, when it has helped define who you are and when you have many memories of highs, friendships, places, and events. As with other disciplines such as music, painting, or hobbies, sports, when we love them, they are like the best relationships. But there are times when we leave them and need something new. Perhaps it's the perfect time to try something new!

Why Change Sports?

The reasons can be many.

• You may just have outgrown the passion for your sport: "Been there, done that". Your interests have changed. You may feel a bit stuck in your life and a new sport would be a way to recharge it. It's easier to change sports than jobs or houses. You want to learn new skills and meet new people.
• You've been injured multiple times in your sport.
• You can't play or compete at the same level.
• Your circumstances change. Maybe you played a team

sport before and there's no comparable team or league in the area. Maybe your family moves and the structure you had disappears.

You've outgrown your passion. It can happen. You loved the sport once and now you want to move on. Maybe you feel burned out. There are so many things in adult life that are hard to change – where you live, what you do, whom you're married to. Why not try a fresh start in something new?

Sue Pevear, now in her fifties, grew up playing tennis. She captained her high school team, played tennis in college, and played on and off after college. For years she thought about getting back to tennis but felt conflicted. She had clearly loved tennis and she still enjoyed it, but it didn't feel like an exciting challenge anymore.

"Many people who take tennis seriously now, did not do it as kids," she said. "They're very focused on it and are able to have the experience of a new high…. so every new peak is a new peak. They are still unfolding in tennis. I feel I have done it and am satisfied with what I've done….Still there was this thought that maybe I should still be playing."

She decided to continue tennis just as a casual sport for socializing, not something to focus on seriously. "Going back to competitive tennis also felt a bit like returning to the past," she said. "Sometimes it's wonderful to return to the past, but sometimes there's also some sadness going back to a sport that meant a lot to me – a sport where the people who had supported me are no longer in my life." Sue has been in her financial management career for decades. A new sport, she felt, would open up a new world for her.

Diane was a dedicated squash player through college and for a number of years after that, until she had children. "Squash is one of those sports that's hard to just pick up. You have to find a facility. You need an opponent --- in fact, you need several. You need to schedule court time. You need to find players whose 'play' schedule matches yours. You also need to be in shape or you'll injure yourself. I love the sport but it just feels too hard to organize so I can't enjoy it the way I used to."

Whatever the sport you've left, however, -- even if you've

moved on – you'll always feel twinges, a yearning, as you watch it. Runners who no longer run will always hear sneakers going by their windows.

<u>You're sick of that same old injury.</u> Bum-mer. How many times can you reinjure yourself – and in the same place? At 38, Sara Weiss finally gave up swimming after the sixth time she injured her rotator cuff. "The decision to stop was tough, so frustrating. I had to come to terms with the fact that my life as a swimmer was over. My thinking kept going around and around in circles as I tried to take a new perspective and figure out how I might do it again. Finally I got fed up with hitting the same wall. I told myself: "Stop complaining. This is just a sport. This isn't my family, my job, or my house…..Still, though, it felt as serious as any of those.

"Leaving swimming was like getting a divorce. My father taught me to swim when I was four. Some of my best friends have been swimmers. Many still are – even though I'm in my late forties now. The thought of leaving swimming felt as if I were cutting myself off from my past – from my old self-image as a strong, young person. But I had to walk away from it."

<u>You can't play at same level.</u> You could, maybe…if you a) were younger b) in better shape c) had more time d) had others you could train with or e), f), g) – whatever they might be. But you are or do not. You wrestle with being a has-been – particularly when you see others your age out there and doing well. "Hey, no fair!" your baby voice cries. On the one hand, you wish for an ideal world without limits – so that you could participate the way you used to.

Anne Epstein enjoyed soccer in high school. "We had so much fun then," she said. "Feeling that sense of belonging regardless of wins or losses gave me a sense of identity that I miss. Now that I work and have a two-year-old, finding a women's soccer team with practices that fit my schedule is too hard. I need to find another activity."

<u>Circumstances change.</u> The logistics don't work for your "old" sport – you move, your work schedule changes, you have children or elderly parents to care for – and the structure that

worked for you evaporates.

Karate enthusiast Karen Roberts had to change sports when her husband's job was relocated from Boston to rural New Hampshire. "We've lived in the Boston area for 15 years, and for the last six I had been taking karate. It felt like getting a new lease on life when I started it. Then we decided we had to move for my husband's career, and my karate world ended. There wasn't a studio nearby in New Hampshire. I felt a major source of my new identity, confidence, and strength disappear."

<u>Letting go.</u> Of all of these situations, the first – the one where you've outgrown the passion – is perhaps the easiest. Moving on is under your control. You are psychologically ready. Once you're ready to change to another sport, think about the guidelines for goals mentioned in Chapter 4 in picking a sport: see the big picture, enter the "beginner's mind", find support, focus your practice, and, remember that mastery takes time.

In the other three scenarios – if you've been injured, if you can't play at the same level, or if your circumstances change – you have to deal with conflicting feelings of leaving your old sport, a sport which was gratifying and fulfilling. While some are able to leave the old anything easily, some of us find it hard to move on when we feel conflicted – in an uncomfortable, in-between place – caught between happy memories of the past, uncertainty about a future direction, indecision in general.

Moving On

Don't get immobilized for too long. (Don't take this too seriously – this is a sport we're talking about here.) So, allow yourself a certain amount of time to process the conflict. "People might say 'it's easy to leave a sport because it's just a sport', but it's you," said masters runner Sue Gustafson. "Many people are accused of being obsessed with their sport. There's a grain of truth in that. You can feel shut out not only of your sport but also of life – of youth and vitality. Your image of success and power are often tied up with your sport in the same way relationships are. In that sense quitting a sport can change your self image the same way losing a relationship can."

Wendy Connelly agrees that leaving a sport is not always a trivial matter. A gymnast through high school, she hasn't been active since then and now it's been about six years. "Being a gymnast is my identity," she said. "Sometimes I feel like I don't care if I ever try any other sport....but other times I feel like I am letting life pass me by. I'm just stuck on that identity and it's silly, but real."

In many cases, you'll know it's time to move on when you start boring yourself by mulling the same thoughts over and over. And don't let yourself fall prey to mere excuses for not moving on!

Steps to help you move on include:

Keeping a journal. Keeping a journal will help you express your feelings about a sport – what you love about it, what hurts about leaving it, how it might help you figure out what to do next. Write a summary of your experience in the sport. At some point you'll get sick of journaling and want to try a new sport.

Sara Weiss started journaling to help her process her life as a swimmer. It helped her ultimately to transition from swimming to soccer.

"For a while – for almost a year – I didn't do much in the way of anything athletic," said Sara. " I tried a few things like jogging and spinning but I was half-hearted about them – totally uninspired. I hadn't 'packaged up' swimming in my head. Until then, I couldn't really make a new plan. I started writing in a journal – just a few words, at most a paragraph. It sounds silly, but it was the 'exercise' that helped me let go of swimming. I wrote about what it meant and about why it was hard to let it go – and then I realized, 'This is stupid! Move on!'....and I did. I got so sick of being stuck in my head that I found something totally different. I'm playing on a women's soccer team now and it's so different and fun."

Meditating or setting aside time daily to sit and think quietly. Karen Roberts meditated. She realized that letting go is not the same as giving up. It can mean "growing". "I realized that, once my children finished high school, which would be in two years,

I would go back to karate," she said. "Meditating helped me realize that. I also realized that I needed something just for me. Meditating helped me turn a 'negative' into a 'positive'. New Hampshire is a great place to bicycle – much better than Boston. It was a great way to enjoy the countryside and stay fit. It was a welcome change from martial arts."

Talking to friends. Talk with others who have also let go of a sport and moved on – or talk with anyone who can talk about moving on from anything from which their identity has been closely tied.

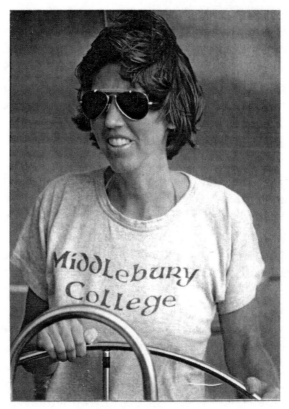

Sue Pevear at the helm.

After talking with friends and playing some casual tennis, former college tennis player Sue Pevear became satisfied that her competitive days were over and has a great time hitting and playing with friends. Talking with others helped her find a new sport which would represent a new challenge in her life – and also a new stage. She realized a new sport would also give her an anchor, a focus that would be something just for her at a time when she was facing many mid-life challenges: a very ill father, mild depression, professional ups and downs, and life as a single woman. So she chose sailing. She sailed a little as a girl – her family had a sunfish – and occasionally she crewed for her uncle.

"I love to be out in nature and remembered that free feeling of being out on the ocean," she said. Sailing was suddenly representative of new life and the future. "It was not like tennis, where I had standards that I had set for myself that were hard to meet.

"With sailing, my excitement and enjoyment were more than I anticipated. I knew I needed something emotionally to help me in life. I was looking forward to being on the ocean, even if I was just sitting on a boat on a mooring. The excitement was to learn about boats, what makes them different (a boat to me was what a bird used to be) – the winds, the weather, the tides…about nature at large. It opened up a subject that was much broader than I thought."

Despite the choice of sailing, Sue still felt somewhat conflicted. "On the one hand, it felt decadent to take the time to do this for myself. On the other hand, I needed it for my self-respect. You're so used to giving everything to everyone else in life or to a job that it was hard in a sense to justify it for myself. But I knew I would feel better if I gave this to myself. It's a problem many women face. Not really knowing whether it was right or wrong, I forged ahead. I said – I have to act – to do something!"

Sue had multiple goals. "Goal #1 was to feel confident taking the boat out into heavy wind and feel I could handle it. Goal # 2 was to get to a point where I could cruise with confidence…to be able to navigate, use a compass, sail out of sight of land…to be able to sail the coast of New England competently… from Maine to Marion to Long Island. And goal #3 was to enjoy a sport that I could enjoy with friends".

While the first and second goals are ones Sue is working on, she has met her third goal. She has enjoyed time with friends and dated several men she's met through sailing.

If you don't want to or can't participate in a sport at the same level, how about coaching it? You may remember Wendy Wilbur, former World Rowing Champion and seven-time U.S. national team member who is now Coaching Assistant for the Radcliffe Crew at Harvard University. She talked about the value of the buddy system in Chapter 6. While she is not a competitor at this point in her life, she has found the rewards of coaching.

"When I was done with my elite rowing career, I took a job in a corporate team building company," she said. "One of the teambuilding exercises that we offered to corporate groups was rowing. We would take professionals out in eight-oared shells, teach them how to row, and then have a race. It was from that job that I realized I was most happy in my job when I was coaching. I have now been coaching for six years and I am fairly sure I have the best job in the world! I take a lot of pride in helping young athletes excel in their sport and feel a definite sense of accomplishment when I see them succeed. My goals become their goals and theirs become mine."

Reframe your perspective on a sport if you want to continue with it but not play on the same level. That's what Sue Pevear did. "Remember your own personal reason for reengaging in that sport. Don't get swept up in the motivations of others around you and lose sight of why you have returned. See yourself through your own eyes and not through others'. This reminds you why you are there – it's about fun."

But, as Sue can attest, there are gains, clearly, from taking up a new sport above and beyond the fact that you learn new skills and make new friends. You learn more about yourself. You learn resilience, flexibility, and resourcefulness.

"You feel young again. It brings you back to an innocence," said Sue. "Everything is new. There is no expectation. The first time you learn to ride a bike you are innocent. You're almost naïve. It gives you energy. It gives freedom and hope."

The beginner's mind can be contagious. Once you dare to leave the familiar and enter a new arena, you meet others who are doing the same – others with an adventurous spirit and open mind. You may realize that change is not as daunting as you might have feared and the energy you derive from it inspires you to think about changes in other areas of life as well. "Cycling has got me thinking about starting a new business career," said Karen.

PART III

Beyond Athletics

Effect of Achieving Athletic Goals on Family

"Call it a clan, call it a network, call it a tribe, call it a family: Whatever you call it, whoever you are, you need one."
- Jane Howard

Athletic goals teach lessons you can apply to family.

You learn patience.

You gain strength and discipline that help you become more assertive and earn greater respect.

You develop closer bonds with family members. You become a role model.

What about the claim on this book's first page that athletic goals can improve your life? I wrote: "It is never too late or too hard to design and achieve a new athletic goal. Achieving that goal can improve your whole life: your career, your relationships, your hobbies, your world." Is that hyperbole? "C'mon," you said, "Improve your whole life?"

Many of us are living the "FR" life. It's frenetic, fragmented, frantic, and frazzled – a dizzying whirlwind of competing responsibilities. First, an athletic goal with its tangible focus serves as a stabilizer, providing a calming perspective amidst the "fr" bluster. How can you strive for a goal without having it affect the rest of your life? The benefits of achieving athletic goals spill over to the rest of life in more ways than can be enumerated – to family, friendships, work, and roles in your community.

The Lessons Of Athletic Goals

If you're pursuing an athletic goal, you can't keep it separate from your family. As you follow your plan, confront challenges, face fears, and overcome obstacles in your sport, you learn tangible lessons from it. The lessons ferment. Your athletic experience helps you respond with more informed wisdom about all kinds of issues. Patience overcoming hurdles in your sport may help you be more patient listening to your child's frustration over chemistry or it may make you a better coach with homework. You may be so used to taking risks that you challenge your partner about his political views. In this chapter, Marianne, Jeanne, and Leni tell how aspects of family life were transformed by their athletic goals.

Patience helps. Marianne T. would not have had children were it not for achieving her athletic goal. Pregnancy was never an option for her. She had had a kidney transplant at 22, endured a three-month stint on dialysis, and taken medications like prednisone ever since to maintain healthy kidney function. However, "Type A" in every respect, she worked long hours for a major Fortune 500 company in real estate – leaving the house at

6:30 a.m. and arriving home at 7:30. "I lived in the 'cubicle world' – on the go 24 by 7," she said. "Of course my husband thought I was working like a maniac," she said. "Sometimes I'd work on my laptop after dinner."

In her mid-thirties, Marianne sought a better life balance. "I didn't want a life dictated 100% by corporate America," she said. "I was lacking Vitamin D and tired of looking at the outside world through my office or car windows." She started exercising, her doctor having recommended moderate weight-bearing exercise. Having been on prednisone since the transplant, she had to avoid exercise that was too stressful on her bones such as running on pavement or hard-impact activities.

Marianne took what she called a "blind leap of faith" when she asked me to be her coach. The concept of making athletic training a priority while balancing a demanding work schedule was new to her. She wanted a coach to help her build an incremental program of biking, weight training, and stretching; to train with her from time to time; to adjust the plan according to her progress and other life events; to encourage her during the inevitable plateaus in training; and to understand all her responsibilities, so that I could help her say "no" to requests for activities that did not represent a priority for her.

"This was so outside my comfort zone," Marianne said. "Starting training and doing something totally non work-related was like going into an unknown world. I didn't even have a bike...or weights, for that matter. I couldn't even bike more than a few minutes at a time, never mind a mile," she said. "Above and beyond the training questions, I was in the habit of saying 'yes' to everything."

Marianne's experience starting from scratch and setting successive short-term goals built confidence in her ability to manage long-term plans. She followed a training schedule of biking four or five times a week, weight training, and stretching, and overcame obstacles like the flu, business trips, and periods of skepticism. She bought a heart rate monitor, weights, the biking gear – the helmet, bike shorts, a weight training book, the bike rack, etc. All of this was completely new to her. She also attended a biking class at the Appalachian Mountain Club to learn how to change a tire and patch a wheel. For several months after work, she drove for an hour to meet me and ride half mile, gradual uphill repeats. She kept a training journal every week during the three years.

Learning patience to follow successive short-term goals, she eventually received medical clearance to set and achieve several long-term goals. She completed two long charity rides, and hiked a number of mountains with her husband and extended family members including Mt. Chocorua and Mt. Kearsage. "If someone had told me a few years before that I had done that, I would have said 'Impossible!'. As a side benefit, we created great beautiful memories hiking with three generations of family members."

Succeeding in an arena far outside her comfort zone, Marianne decided she was ready to work hard for something she had always dismissed as being too difficult: adopting a child. Pursuing biking and hiking goals had taught her patience – to commit to a process, to divide a long-term goal into small steps, and to persevere through unexpected hurdles. All those lessons helped during the two-year adoption process.
"It was revolutionary for us to have a child – a blind leap of faith. I felt I was jumping off a cliff into a new life to break the bonds of the work force. You cover your eyes and just jump, not knowing know what's on the other end. It felt like a windy, twisty road of unknowns…but it was similar to my experience training."

The patience and faith in attention to detail she gained from her biking experience helped her face and overcome the many details and obstacles inherent in adopting. "We had to collect photos for an album, obtain references, write essays for applications, and participate in many interviews," she said. "The paperwork itself is a long, arduous task."

The adoption process itself took several years with unexpected delays. Marianne recalled, for example, that, ten months after starting the process, she and her husband were approved for adoption. Five months after that, they were one of two couples selected by a birth mother to adopt her unborn child. "It was down to two people with the choice in the hands of the birth mother who only knew us through a photo album and essays as she was in college and out of town ," said Marianne. "We thought why wouldn't she pick us? We are active, committed, and young – but not too young and we have large, nice, involved local families'. Anyway, we did not get the final nod. She picked the other couple."

Why?

"You have to put together a photo journal, and the birth mother picked the other couple because, one, she liked the other couple's boat – it reminded her of her childhood and two, she liked the Christmas tree in the others' journal. When you hear those arbitrary reasons, you say 'what?' Then you think 'Should I pursue this? This is really disappointing.' But then I realized that, somewhat like my biking and hiking goals, I had a goal to meet. It was disappointing to be declined but we wanted a child and wanted to adopt and we were going to pursue it. So we continued to wait."

And wait. Three months later they were chosen again, and this time the baby became theirs. Marianne ended up leaving her job to be a full-time mother and wife, while also volunteering for various local non-profit charities. "I would never trade my time for money ever again," she said. "I have no remorse leaving corporate America in the rear view mirror. Our life is so much healthier and fulfilling beyond belief. I am so grateful to have a beautiful son. He is a gift from God – a 100% gift. What a shame if I was still adding up numbers in a column to try to make a real estate deal work. I'd rather watch my son score a goal in a hockey net, get high honors, grow into a size 6 shoe, or fall into our dishwasher while moon dancing…the way he did last night! I wouldn't want to miss that joy."

Respect and Self-Discipline. Who needs to be reminded that teens are a challenge? Teens are even challenging for professionals whose career is focused on children through the teenage years. Meet Jeanne Benjamin, pediatrician and psychotherapist. "Raising children, and particularly teens, is no easy task," said Jeanne.

As a wife and mother in her thirties and early forties, she tried to be nurturing, selfless, and accommodating. "I had been raised to be a good wife and mother which meant adapting to my husband's and children's needs – otherwise I would be selfish." She was compliant about exercise, too. "My husband wanted to run," she said. "So I started to run– to be an agreeable mate. But," she said, "I hated running. It was so boring. Then I tried aerobics and jazzercise. I did free weights and Nautilus. It was mindless." None of these activities sparked her interest. Working and taking care of her husband and three children, she often felt depleted.

In helping her son sign up for a martial arts class, Jeanne unwittingly found she had stumbled – at 45 – on a new activity that would become her passion. "I wanted to help teach him the moves," she said. Moo Do, a Korean martial art, became not only an activity for her son but also a passion for Jeanne. "Growing up, I was not the athlete. While I never feared anything intellectually, it made me nervous to compete physically," she said. While she took dance from elementary school through college, she said "I grew up at a time when it wasn't ladylike to compete physically. I graduated from high school in 1968 and in P.E. we wore the bloomers."

Her new athletic endeavor transformed her life, from the inside out. "Something clicked. This is an old style of martial arts. There's a protocol for everything. You bow to your instructors. Those dudes were like Bruce Lee. They could *move!* I had been a 'don't-tell-me-what-to-do' person so I was training my mind in new way."

Loving the exacting discipline, she started training as many as 20 hours a week. "I was fortunate that my husband works so I did not to have to work full-time and could be in control of my hours," she said. During weekday mornings she worked as a therapist. She attended a noon class and then, two nights a week, took a two to three hour class. "Learning Moo Do ain't fast," she said. The challenges of the discipline include hundreds of movement patterns, each with its own name – like Pal Gae – and its own precise sequence of multiple twists, kicks, punches, turns, bends, sweeps, and strikes. "During classes – and some can be two and a half hours long, you have instructors walking around, telling you specifically what to do, such as 'Get down low! Get that knee straight! Get that arm up!'

"The precision of your position reflects the power and movement of Chi, an energy that is part of the physical world and that martial artists learn how to circulate in and out of the body so both body and mind function better and with more force. A martial arts master cycles Chi energy all the time," she said. "You learn the power of Chi – it takes time to master." Her husband started Moo Do as well.

As a result of Chung Moo Do, Jeanne not only improved her stamina, power, and flexibility (she can still palm the ground with both hands) but also became more assertive with her family. "Moo Do showed me that I have some power in my life. It reinforced and supported a sense of myself as an active player – that I don't have to let things just happen in life and suffer the consequences – and it gave me permission to take care of myself," she said.

She became more energetic and positive with her family. "I learned that if you're putting energy out, you need to put some energy in. Learning to articulate my needs was helpful for my husband and kids. I realized I need to take time for myself: that I am not an unending well of love and compassion, giving and understanding – all that good stuff. Many women feel badly about themselves for not being a bottomless well of caring. They want to do more and more for others and get more and more depressed. Depression is a system of depletion."

She carried her body more assertively, earning more respect from her husband and teenagers. She had more authority. "I was raised traditionally – in a 'Father Knows Best Household,'" she said. "With Moo Do, I became a powerful woman in their eyes. There's a physical change that's visible to everyone. You carry your body differently. You get taller. You don't slump your shoulder. Your chest is open. You stand upright." she said. "My family saw a woman who is powerful – just by how I carried my body – not a weak, vulnerable woman. That engenders respect.

"My children are proud of me even though they didn't go down that path," said Jeanne. "You don't see the seeds you sew right away. They all know that being physically fit is something I value, and they are active in other ways." Though none of them practices Moo Do, Jeanne's children all value exercise, and they report their activities to Jeanne. "They still care about what I think. One will say 'You know? I went running today.' Or 'we went hiking and roller blading.'"

The Power of A Role Model. You met Leni Webber earlier in this book – in Chapter 7 as she discussed overcoming injuries and in Chapter 8 as she told about overcoming personal and professional setbacks. At 49, Leni asked me to help her to pursue running goals and, specifically, to get faster and feel stronger. An insurance advisor, wife, and mother, Leni felt that weekly coaching would provide consistency, accountability, and support – 'CAS' as she calls it – that would help her reach her potential. "I had run throughout my 30s and considered myself a fairly good runner….but I wasn't consistent and I hadn't set goals. I thought I might do better, and balance everything else if I had someone help me set goals while considering everything else going on in life. I wanted to set other life goals as well."

She wanted help with training plans and choosing races and also support – particularly as she was in her late forties, when others have given up on their athletic goals. "For older people starting things," Leni said, "it's very hard to see the incremental progress if you're doing it by yourself because there are too many other competing priorities." Leni worked with me on planning and scheduling her workouts and also on managing work responsibilities so they did not conflict with her athletic goals. In her case, she focused on not booking sales appointments at times when she had planned to run. "Having someone say 'you will age better with training' and reminding me that I would improve over time – ten years, 10,000 hours – helped me stay focused on my goals and appreciate the incremental progress," she said.

Incremental progress she has made. Despite injuries, she has improved steadily over the past 15 years. With the additional support of her husband, Alan, she has run short and long races and participated in biking events and triathlons. In her early sixties, she ran her best 5K race relative to her age after 12 years of training. "My race results have been extremely gratifying because I have seen my hard work pay off."

Perhaps the most rewarding aspect of Leni's experience achieving her running goals is that they ultimately bonded her with her teenage son, Ben. As mentioned in Chapter 8, Ben had – like many teenagers – experienced academic and social challenges. He felt apathetic, even hopeless, about school and athletics. He left the public school to attend a private school in Maine. There, at 17, he joined the cross country and track teams. Being on the teams presented a challenge at first. He was concerned about not meeting others' expectations. "At one point the coach didn't feel as if he was running up to his potential," said Leni.

Ben had seen Leni's success from persistence and consistency and ultimately displayed both, which helped his running. "His breakthrough in running went hand in hand with his breakthrough in his emotional growth – and he also had a role model," said Leni. "When your mother goes out and runs at 6 a.m. in 10 degrees consistently...when you cheer your mother on in a half marathon...you know her values."

Ben got faster and faster. His cross country team won the state championships in its division and the team competed in the Regional Junior Olympics. The team then qualified for the National Junior Olympics. "He now sees himself as a winner," said Leni. He just won the award for the most determined athlete on the cross country team and he has been named its captain. "He is now a leader in his school, a role model for others. He is researching colleges that offer majors in business and computer science."

How would she describe the bond between them?

"We both have a bond in the joy of excelling and being a member of a team. We know what it's like to push beyond what one thinks one is capable of."

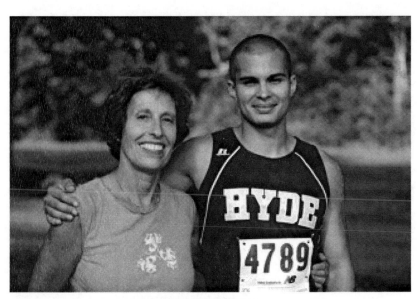

Ben and Leni Webber

12

The Effect of Achieving Athletic Goals on Friends

"A friend is someone who understands your past, believes in your future, and accepts you just the way you are."
- Unknown

Great friendships are forged through sweat.

Athletic friends can come to feel like family when goals are shared.

Unexpected friendships arise from pursuing athletic goals.

Friendships, new and old, are enriched through shared athletic goals.

What woman – single, divorced, widowed, or married – doesn't want good friendships? Pursuing athletic goals affects the nature of friendships in countless ways. It can lead to new friendships and create new avenues of growth for long-time friendships.

Friends make achievements more meaningful. What is a success without being able to share it with friends? Our friends help us enjoy and see the unique meaning of our achievements. They know the challenges we have to overcome. They know why we want to test ourselves. We hope that they will, in turn, take on challenges that have meaning for them.

At the same time, when we fall short of our vision of ultimate achievement, we have others beside us, our athletic partners who sense and value our willingness to see our imperfections. Because athletic partners grow in their trust of each other, these friendships allow the giving and receiving of thoughts and feelings much more than in our normal daily interactions with others. We support each other in times of success and failure and all of us highly value that support. It strengthens the bonds of our friendships and, in many cases, these friendships become timeless.

In the following three stories, Bethany, Lisa, and Beth and Rose tell what they gained from athletic goals that affected their friendships and their lives in general. They are not intended to be representative of all women's stories, necessarily; there are as many stories as there are women.

A Feeling Of Belonging

"It doesn't always feel great to be single in your mid-thirties. You can feel left out," said Bethany Edwards. Now married, she was single through her twenties and thirties. It wasn't easy.
A runner whom I coach and a member of the Liberty Athletic Club, Bethany said she would be happy to share her thoughts on how athletic goals helped her as a woman when she was single. "It's scary to be single when a majority of your friends have established families and stable partners. You're thinking that you've failed. Why haven't I done what I am supposed to do as a woman? Why

haven't I established that home, that relationship hopefully for the rest of my life? What did I do wrong?"

"We're all searching for stability. When you're single, that stability of what a woman is expected to have – a husband, 2.5 kids, a nice house, and dinner on the table every night. If that 1950s homemaker lifestyle isn't there, you have to search for stability in other areas of life. Many of us have that stability at work but once you leave work you wonder 'What do I do now?'"

Bethany had these thoughts even though she led a full life. She worked 9:30 to 6:30 p.m., five days a week as a managing editor at the Milford Daily, a local community newspaper that covers 12 towns in Massachusetts. Outside work, she taught three to five year olds in Sunday school ("we basically play"), and spent time with friends. A 400 meter runner in college, she continued to run after college, occasionally entering road races.

Sensing that she needed a boost, I suggested that Bethany "buddy-up" with Sue Gustafson, a Liberty Athletic Club runner who is more than 20 years older than Bethany. "Having a buddy in Sue was inspiring," said Bethany. "First, she's an awesome runner – and a great person. Second, working as a team and communicating even if just by e-mail every week created a feeling of focus, belonging, and stability that was powerful." The MOVE! buddy system also helped Bethany overcome the four main obstacles she had identified – "the fear of her hip injury returning, not making her time goals, occasionally feeling unmotivated, and struggling through every run."

"Friendship is huge when you don't have that boyfriend or partner. You turn to your girlfriends as your stable social outlook. I think those girlfriends for a single girl tend to become deeper in your late twenties and thirties when you have time to devote to them -- deeper than in your teens and early twenties. They (girlfriends) are sort of like family for you."

She took up triathlon at 32 for several reasons. First, she said, "I wanted a new challenge." Swimming and biking were new for her. "I'm a lousy swimmer. I had swimming lessons in elementary school but I never swam between that and the triathlon. I played around in the ocean but never got in a pool and did laps. Swimming requires form, so I had to do repeat drills in the pool. Biking was the same. Everyone has a bike as a kid but I never biked for distance."

Second, she was looking for a kind of commitment that was significant and personal – the kind she missed in not having her own family. The commitment involved in having to show up for early morning workouts with a group of other women gave her the sense of belonging and community that she missed.

"When you create that extra piece – in this case, athletics – it gives you another stable group you can focus on. You have work, and then you have this group of women and a 'buddy' that gives that stability outside of work that you may not have. You develop solid friendships." Knowing that I had to show up to meet a group of women to train every week on Wednesdays and Saturdays gave me and others a commitment and feeling of belonging. There were several times on Wednesdays after work when I was too tired but I knew that, if I didn't go, the others would know. I couldn't let these people down. I needed to show up. They were counting on me.

"Constant commitment is a level of responsibility. You don't ever want to break month-long plans with friends. To train for an event, you are making a promise to yourself and these other women that you are someone who can be counted on to finish the goal. There's not the same level of promise if you arrange to go to the movies. The connection with others going for the same goal is satisfying in a way that occasional connections are not."

Unexpected Friendships

Lisa is a competitive golfer who came to me to help her set specific deliberate practice goals to improve her game. (She lowered her handicap significantly in only six weeks.) Her story illustrates the unexpected friendships one gains from setting athletic goals. She took up golf seriously in her late thirties, having played as a girl and not liked it. "Ironically I started liking it when I finished grad school and no longer had access to a course."

The chief financial officer of an investment company, she wanted help joining a country club where she could play. "The only thing I ever asked my boss was to help me join a country club. I knew no one who played. My boss found me two sponsors and, in my late thirties, I joined a golf club." She started playing on week-ends, often every week.

She clearly "caught the passion". In her forties, Lisa was financially able to retire and focus even more intensely on a goal. She was most comfortable on the golf course. "Every morning when I would drive to the club and see the club's picket fence, my heart would start beating faster. I'd think, 'Oh yay, I get to go hit golf balls'.

"I would be out on the range by myself hour after hour, trying to get better and trying to improve my swing and people would come up on the course and introduce themselves. I was really surprised because I am uncomfortable at parties and cocktail parties...but meeting people on the range was very easy because we had something in common – our love of golf."

Starting in 2003, Lisa's involvement in competitive club golf intensified as she started taking lessons and playing club tournaments. "My pro encouraged me to play in competitions and that brought me into another small group within the club -- the women who played in competitions. With those women I had something in common: the competitive fire. Those friendships were comfortable because even though we competed against and with each other, we shared so much including how nervous you get before competitions, etc."

In 2005, she started playing in state competitions. Eventually she was asked to be president of her country club's women's golf association. "As president, I tried to play with every woman member. I met tons of women. It was wonderful," she said. Then she was asked to join the board of the Women's Golf Association of Massachusetts (WGAM), a 110-year-old organization that runs all women's state golf tournaments.

"Through that, I met lots of other people including the best women golfers in the state. It was really fun. I was so impressed with how willing these women are to share what they know...I mean, I am competing against them and they're still so generous with their knowledge."

Recently, at an awards ceremony hosted by the WGAM at her country club, Lisa realized how important her golf friendships have become, even though she didn't get into golf to build her friendships. "I was not going to go to the ceremony. But then I did, and I realized how much I belonged and how many friends I had. Someone hugged me when I arrived and immediately introduced me to someone new. I knew so many people there and I knew everyone on the board. I thought 'This is my tribe'.

"All of this came as a complete surprise. I never thought of joining the board at WGAM, of competing in state tournaments, of being on the board at my club. I never thought about making new friends and acquaintances. It came completely unplanned as I focused so much on getting better at golf."

Recently, Lisa welcomed a new member to her club. "I told her she ought to play in some state tournaments and she said, "Oh – will you be my mentor?"

Good Friendships Become Richer

In their sixties, Beth Steffian and Rose Ashby had been living full lives (high powered careers – Beth, a management consultant and Rose, a Harvard Ph.D. and college president) and had no intention of slowing down. They were colleagues who hired me in tandem – first one, then the other. They had grown up before colleges offered many, if any, sports for women, and they wanted help in figuring out what physical achievements might suit their interests (running was not one of them), strengths (endurance, patience, curiosity) and weaknesses (they were not in their twenties). They were game to apply the *MOVE!* method. OK, I said, take your time to think of goals that have meaning for you. The *MOVE!* Athletic Options Form was helpful. So was time.

Beth and Rose just knew that they wanted to be strong. "If you're going to stay young," said Rose, "you have to stay moving and active. I always have dreams of places I want to go. I've always loved to walk.

"I was approaching the end of my career and looking for some big project to undertake – I didn't want to resort to alcohol or put my nose in a book 24 hours a day," said Beth. "We both liked walking," said Rose. "We could do something long. We liked the idea of setting a goal and conquering a distance."

At one point, Beth came up with the goal of hiking after reading Bill Bryson's, <u>A Walk in the Woods.</u> "My great inspiration was Bill Bryson. He sends a Christmas card and says 'Does anyone want to come with me?' I put out an SOS.... I started asking all my friends who might have a faint interest. I sent them copies of this wonderful book published by the Sierra Club."

Rose was the first one to join, along with another friend from work, Carlyn. Beth also enlisted a friend from college days, Charlotte, and another friend, Kitsie, whom she had known from her early married days. "Everyone was fascinated by the idea." The group ranged in age from late fifties to early sixties. "It was interesting. We didn't all know one another. It took a couple of weeks to work out the kinks – to sort out everyone's likes and dislikes. We never really did become a close knit hiking group, but we developed wonderful friendships that bridged other parts of our lives, and brought many unexpected pleasures."

Their initial goal was the Camino de Santiago de Compostela (The Way of St. James), the oldest pilgrimage trail in Europe. There are many starts (e.g., Brittany, Paris, Provence). The routes all meet in the Pyrenees and go west, crossing through Spain and ending near the Atlantic coast at Santiago de Compostela.

The five women hiked the first week together through the Pyrenees. "It was very steep," said Rose. "Some days you are on country roads, gravel, dirt roads, minor asphalt roads," said Beth, who has hiked since all over Europe, including Corsica, Scotland, and three weeks in the Soviet Union in the Caucasus Mountains. "Some days you are scrambling up hills. Some days you descend a rocky path in the mud and you think your knees will go out before you get there. You traverse rocks, mud, mountain tops, roots.

"We stayed in little one-star hotels, sometimes better and sometimes worse," said Rose. "We carried what we needed for the day. Some days we had terrible weather – at some points we were clomping around mud that was knee deep with five pounds of mud stuck to our boots. We were soaked....anyway, we had a wonderful time. The scenery was beautiful with Roman bridges, wonderful forests, charming villages, and little Romanesque churches... the path is a miracle, architecturally – because it grew

up along this famous pilgrimage that even Charlemagne took."
How did it affect their friendships? They've become fuller. "One of
the unexpected pleasures of this kind of walking/hiking/trekking
has been the friendships along the way - both with those in the
group, and those we met outside of it," said Beth. "In Scotland,
I walked with an old college friend with whom I hadn't had any
quality time for years. We have shared a lot of pain, and learned
to tolerate it.

"You get to know one another in ways that you don't
typically know your friends. You look for the person who doesn't
give out under pressure and fatigue. You get a very good sense of
people's strengths and weaknesses that you don't ordinarily see
in friendship. You spend eight hours walking with someone and
then you spend the night nursing your body and you get to know
people very well.

"We do support one another off the trail," said Beth. "One
of us has become seriously ill in the last year and we have all pulled
together to support her – and it has brought us together as a group
so that now we do things together in a different way – that isn't
hiking. For instance, it is difficult for our sick member to travel

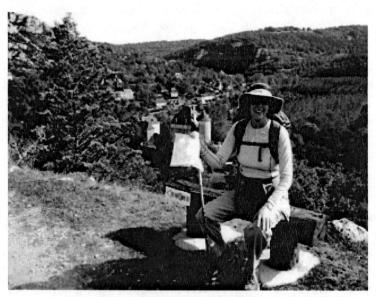

Rose Ashby hiking the Camino de Santiago de Compostela
(The Way of St. James) in southwestern France.

so we are bringing her a meal. One of us has a daughter who is getting married this summer and she has invited everyone to the wedding events. We will all see one another. We have supported one another's children with job applications."

"Long distance walking has changed the rhythm of our lives," said Rose. "Every few months I get itchy. My husband, John, cannot believe me as a 70-year old lady tearing up these hills. He can't believe how I can zip up and down all these slopes. He is flabbergasted. So am I. We are so much stronger and more capable physically than we ever thought we could be."

13

Effect of Achieving Athletic Goals on Work

"The dog that trots about finds a bone."
- George Henry Borrow

Goal setting and achievement are as essential to work as they are to athletics.

Athletic goals must be concrete. Achievement of your athletic goals shows you can apply MOVE! to work goals. Once you've achieved your athletic goal, it's easy to apply the MOVE! method to work.

> • *Achieving athletic goals can give you confidence to change career direction, and enhance employee productivity and morale.*
> • *MOVE! may even inspire you to restructure your office completely.*

Thoughts about our athletic goals follow us wherever we go. We succeed in getting through a tough period of training in our sport and, all of a sudden, a tough period at work may feel surmountable. Achieving an athletic goal can spur us on to achieve work goals. Athletic goals are tangible; we can see the concrete results. Athletic settings are often more clear-cut and less complicated than work settings. Achieving an athletic goal is particularly convincing since we know we, individually, were responsible for achieving them – unlike achievements in other more complicated areas of life where there are more factors or players involved. We believe firmly in ourselves when we've achieved an athletic goal.

In this chapter, three women tell how their experiences of setting athletic goals with the *MOVE!* method helped them use the same process with different aspects of their work lives. For Sarah, an athletic goal became an anchor that gave her courage to test the waters and make a transition from a secure career to a new work interest. Setting athletic goals helped Dr. Julie Burke set goals at work. Dr. Barbara Stewart applied the patience she learned in achieving her running goals to restructuring her medical practice and installing a new medical records system. Your experience with athletic and work goals may well be very different from theirs. Again, there are an infinite number of stories that apply. But here are a few which are common in my experience.

An Anchor During A Career Transition

Life can be tough during a career transition – particularly one when you're leaving work you've had for years and when that work has been inextricable from family. Work was family for Sarah. She worked in a family business – a nursery – for over ten years, and when she wanted to move on to develop her own interests, it was an athletic goal that helped ease the transition.

"We were the typical tight-knit, immigrant family which starts a business that employs a few people in the family from each generation," said Sarah. Her grandparents came over from Holland to open the nursery in the early 1930s. When Sarah finished high school at 18, she began working there, interested both in plants and in human resources. "When I graduated from high school in the 1990s, jobs were scarce and I thought I would be able to learn as much at the nursery as at any other job. I jumped at the opportunity of a job there during the summer after high school and just stayed," she said. "I wasn't ready for college when September came around."

In her mid-twenties she met her husband when he came to the nursery as a sales representative for a seed company. "We had a lot in common, both knowing the nursery business – and the rest is history." Married a year later, the couple had a son two years after that.

Managing ten employees, Sarah enlarged the company, adding product lines from bird feeders to wind chimes to books and building a reputation for one of the finest nurseries in the area. In addition to working 60 or more hours a week, she raised her son and was active in her town's gardening club. "It was all-consuming – satisfying on the one hand, but I never had any time to think outside the box. I was on a treadmill, and had to keep moving."

In her early 30s, after more than 12 years in the business, in her early 30s, Sarah felt she wanted some time for herself, including time to get in shape. "Yes – I overworked," she said. "I'd be at the nursery on Saturday nights when my friends were out for dinner and I'd be there on holidays from dawn to dusk. At the end of holidays I'd be beaten up." Sarah barely had time to plan Thanksgiving dinners – one of her favorite pastimes. She had put on 20 extra pounds over the years and envied other women running in the streets. "I wanted to run," she said. "I wanted to be a participant, not an observer. I had never allowed myself time for just me."

Just before her 32nd birthday, Sarah decided to become serious about achieving an athletic goal. She asked me to help her. "I'm not the real athletic type, and I had always thought that, if I wasn't going to be the best, then why bother doing this? But I was intrigued about the *MOVE!* method and setting athletic goals. I thought it would help me get in shape, make time for myself, and explore my own values," she said.

While she started by jogging 30 seconds at a time, Sarah persisted each week. Her first six week goal was to jog for 20 consecutive minutes and lift weights two to three times a week. She kept records and continued to set six-week goals and became an athlete, running several five and ten kilometer races. She lost 17 pounds.

Her greatest achievement was a mini-triathlon, involving a 3.1 mile run, a 15 mile bike ride, and a one third mile ocean swim. The swimming part of the triathlon was daunting for her, someone who usually began by hyperventilating every time she put her face in the pool. Swimming lessons and persistence helped. "I was so afraid of the swim," she said. "And yet I knew I had to learn to deal with my fears and move through them." Sarah completed the mini-triathlon, "the most emotional and exciting event I ever did. It was a gold medal in my mind. I showed up for myself and faced my worst fear."

Success with athletic events – and particularly the mini-triathlon – gave her confidence to face another unknown: to leave the family business and think about a new career. Sarah had used the *MOVE!* forms to set goals and track her athletic progress. Why not use them for her career goals? She got a notebook just to write down her thoughts about her career, and reread what she wrote each week. "I applied the step by step experience of setting athletic goals to setting professional goals." On a Short-Term Goal form she noted the following goals: "1) Make a date with self to go on a soul searching mission 2) Stop looking back - walk forward and face the fears ahead 3) It's ok not to know exactly what I want to do – accept the uncertainty of what's ahead 4) It doesn't have to all feel good. 5) Accept a sense of loss 6) Read books about transitions and 7) Have patience."

Reading books about transitions – including Overwhelmed: Coping with Life's Ups and Downs [18] and Transitions: Making Sense of Life's Changes [19] – helped her a great deal. From the latter

18. Schlossberg, Overwhelmed.

19. William Bridges, Transitions: Making Sense of Life's Changes (Cambridge, MA: Da Capo Press, 2004).

book, she realized she couldn't make a career transition without enduring what the author, William Bridges, calls "the neutral zone". That's an in-between place where you have left your past but haven't stepped into the next spot, a place of uncertainty and turmoil. First, with encouragement from her husband, she decided she did want to get a college degree. "It's hard to go through the uncertainties of transitions, but having weekly goals and writing them down in a notebook helps you see that you are moving ahead – even though it feels slow."

Sarah moved ahead. She is now in her third year on her way to getting her bachelor's degree at the University of Massachusetts, majoring in education and human development. "At the rate I'm going it may take me two more years just to get my undergraduate degree and I'm thinking of getting a masters in social work after that. I'm on the long-term plan. I keep remembering ten years, 10,000 hours to excellence."

She hasn't "arrived" at her next step yet, but she is on her way.

Applying *MOVE!* To The Workplace

The experience of setting athletic goals helped chiropractor Dr. Julie Burke set professional goals that resulted in a restructuring of the way her company operated. In her late twenties, Dr. Burke became the sole proprietor of an holistic health center. In her early thirties, Julie hired me for a variety of reasons. She was working long hours – often 60 a week managing ten employees including four chiropractors, a nutritionist, two massage therapists, and administrative staff. A gymnast and 400 meter sprinter in high school, she wanted to stay in shape and thought that setting some running goals would help her preserve some time for herself, keep her work life in perspective, and get in better shape than attending classes at the gym. "I wanted not just to stay in shape but train for goals and balance my practice as well. I knew goals would help me be more focused, and a coach would ensure that I'd be accountable for my plans," she said.

She embraced the *MOVE!* method and we sat down to

set her goals. Over a two month period we worked on the Three Month Calendar, the Big Picture Calendar, the Short-Term Goal, the Annual Goal, the Three Month Calendar and the Buddy Discussion, all of which helped her set out the athletic, personal, and professional obligations for the year and decide which were most important and which were merely distractions. By the end of the two-month period, she could tell that the goals on her forms were ones she was committed to. "I could look at the whole year – everything. Before even choosing a goal, I could check the dates of conferences, seminars, continuing education courses, and also any plans with my family. I have to travel a lot, so trips are a challenge. Looking ahead gave a birds-eye perspective to see the better months for training and the better week-ends for competing." After setting year-long goals with the *MOVE!* method, she set successive six-week short-term goals.

While there were weeks when not all goals were accomplished – and that will inevitably happen – weekly coaching helped her be accountable and achieve most of them. "Sometimes it took me longer to get to my goal but being accountable every week I had to face it and continue with it." She still remembers surpassing a goal as one of her highest achievements. She wanted to race the mile in 6:15, and she ran it in 6:09.

About six years after setting athletic goals, Julie started implementing the *MOVE!* method at work. "I realized that the office had been operating amidst craziness," she said. "I realized that all my enthusiasm and passion for my practice had to get reined in to be effective – that it had been creating chaos. I would have great expectations in terms of what we could do, but they weren't realistic and never managed."

Unrealistic expectations at the office hurt her self-esteem. "I felt like a failure because I would measure myself against the best, without my own athletic process of goal setting where I'd set goals based on where I was. Instead, I used to look at the most successful practices and think we should be able to do that. It's as if you are a beginning model and think you have to look as good as Christie Brinkley...or a fairly new competitive swimmer who has to swim as fast as Mark Spitz. Setting athletic goals taught me to set goals based on me. It became a habit to stop and ask 'What is realistic?' Goal setting using the *MOVE!* method helped me manage my expectations and become more realistic about time. It also kept a feeling of painful failure at bay. I knew from running that success in achieving goals led to more success."

Julie implemented aspects of *MOVE!* for both the office as a whole and for individual employees. At first, she said, her employees resisted the idea of setting goals. Some were worried that they wouldn't be able to perform. Then they realized the benefits of having tangible goals.

"We would all sit down in December and think about major priorities for the office as a whole. I have a year-long calendar in the employee lounge. It's an erasable board that has all major company projects. I show annual goals on this calendar to my staff so they know when we will implement new systems. If we write in a project for six months ahead, it makes them feel calm, and stops nervous chatter, because they know when their role in the project takes place. It also gives me credibility and helps everyone prepare mentally for the future." Julie works with each employee to determine individual, four-week goals for frequent reinforcement and accountability. "I give them an acceptable range for a goal and I ask them to pick what their goal is."

Julie's goal-setting process using the *MOVE!* method has improved office productivity and morale. Profits have risen every year since instituting the goal setting system. "Productivity is the basis of morale. The numbers help make good performers feel more secure about their jobs. If people are successful in meeting their goals, they get excited. It's contagious."

Julie gave an example of how the *MOVE!* goal setting method for her business made her pay more attention to the financial end of the business. "After checking the numbers I learned a startling truth. I found an employee had cheated the office and falsified reports," she said. "The employee's job was to collect from the insurance companies. "Instead of figuring out how to collect the money she would write off the balance – losing me thousands of dollars. She'd print out patient statements and put them in the dumpster. The process of goal setting forced me to look at the numbers, find the truth, and correct the problem."

Julie is now confident that with tangible short- and long-term goals she can overcome almost any office challenge. "I've learned persistence," she said. "Along the way all kinds of frustrating, discouraging issues come up -- staff issues, changes in insurance law, etc. Goals make you ask 'Are you on the right path? Can you do it?' Goals remind you that your focus is still ahead. You shouldn't get stuck looking at that barrier that's right in your face. You may say "agh... aghhhh" but then you move forward. Even if you don't quite hit the goal, you've still moved forward in the right direction."

Courage To Rebuild A Business

For years, internist Dr. Barbara Stewart had a standard medical practice. Divorced at 31, she had worked hard to raise two children on her own. She had started medical school in her late twenties when her son and daughter were four and seven, respectively. She so wanted to be a doctor then that she worked extremely long hours, sometimes 36 hours in a row. "I had a live-in nursing student. I exchanged room and board for child care to help with the kids and sometimes they were with their father," she said. After graduating at age 38, she started in a traditional medical practice. She loved the work and her practice grew over a period of 19 years. The "downside" was that she had many patients, the hours were very long, and she actually found it hard to make ends meet.

"I was terribly overworked to the point of exhaustion and also underpaid," she said. "I was working 80 to 100 hours a week and earning hardly enough to make a mortgage payment. The trouble was that, if I took the time to listen to people's problems, I couldn't see enough patients in the day to make ends meet. The more time I took with patients, the less money I made. At the same time, I was unable to participate in normal life events. I didn't have as much time as I would have liked to be with my children. I was missing their ball games and some school functions. I wasn't able to go out to see friends in the evening." She even had little time to talk on the phone with family. In short, she said, "my satisfaction was hugely diminished."

Throughout the years, she kept in shape by running races. She recalls that she learned a major lesson after her first race – a lesson that she kept relearning. "When I did my very first race ever, I was afraid of the unknown...that I might find it really stressful. But it wasn't. I was very surprised."

Barbara came to me, having heard about *MOVE!* from Dr. Nina Carroll, a fellow medical doctor. "Nina had said she had a schedule and a program. It seemed to me that *MOVE!* was putting a more intellectual and planned schedule to exercise than I currently had. The casual racing was fun but this was something very different. There was a body of knowledge about training, physiology, and habits that was applied to exercise to which I had not been privy. It was a motivating way to attain goals."

Athletic goals, she said, have helped her build faith in her ability to handle the unknown and succeed despite whatever challenges lie ahead. This faith, she said, was critical in setting a career goal that was frightening at the onset. The goal was to restructure her practice: to change it from being a standard medical to a concierge practice, one where people pay an annual fee to be part of a company which arranges membership in the practice.

Barbara's fears were great and specific. "I was concerned that my patients might be disappointed, that the community would feel I let them down, that I would be seen as money grubbing, and most importantly, that I had had a dedication to my patients which I couldn't continue," she said. "They had a choice – contributing some money to the practice or finding medical care elsewhere. It was frightening to think about changing relationships that I had had for so many years. I was afraid I was going to sink the whole enterprise and moreover I had a huge amount of grief over any relationship that ended in this way.

"However, I have learned from all the athletic challenges that no matter how great the fear, or how big the event, or how important, that I need to employ the same skills to deal with it. I have found that once I talk something through and think about it, I lose the fear. In this situation, it was a mixture of fear and pain. For example, I was talking about the restructuring two or three years before I was able to effect the plan, and I knew I was able to follow through with it because of the experience and success I had making athletic plans and realizing them."

Barbara's fears of not being able to build a viable practice were unjustified, despite the sadness of losing patients. "I had a hard time even looking at charts of patients who did not continue with me, " she said, adding that "about 15 to 20% of my patients stayed, the average percentage when a doctor makes this kind of change. I felt sad about losing patients, but they understood and now I have a practice that I can maintain. With this concierge practice I have a somewhat normal life – just 50 to 60 hours a week, and make enough money to pay my mortgage and I have time to be involved with the lives of my children, grandchildren, and friends. The income from this is far more than I could make under the old system." Her practice has a waiting list now.

Effect of Achieving Athletic Goals on Community

"Act as if what you do makes a difference. It does."
- William James

MOVE! goal setting strategies apply to most things in life, including our communities and the larger world.

Achievement in sports with MOVE! can give you the confidence to volunteer, fundraise, and lead an organization or volunteer effort.

Is it a stretch to think of our athletic goals as having an effect on our communities and the larger world? Not at all. When we strive for athletic goals, we practice dreaming; when we begin our training, we envision a stronger self and imagine the challenges ahead. It's not a stretch to equate a goal with a dream, particularly if the goal is a long-term one. In achieving athletic goals, we realize athletic dreams and have concrete proof, in general, that realizing other dreams in other areas of life is possible.

The World Can Open Up

Pam Kunkemueller was widowed young, at 58. Her husband Jim died at 59 after a nine year struggle with an Alzheimer's related disease. Over those nine years, Pam took care of him "24/7"; first, at home with increasing outside help, and then for the last two years, in a nursing home. Along the way, she says, they learned more about living and loving than they ever had before.

Facing life alone after Jim's death was a major adjustment. Pam had spent most of her adult life as a full-time mother of two and then a full-time caretaker. She had been fully focused on the needs of her family. When she suddenly had to face life alone, she was exhausted, out of shape, and unsure of what to do next. Her children were grown. What should she do with her time? She wasn't used to having any.

"After Jim died, I realized that for the first time in my life I could do whatever I chose to do," she said. "I no longer had to think about anybody else -- not my parents, my sister, my husband, or my children. I didn't have even vague ideas of what my activities might be. I could talk about things that were wrong, but had no clear vision of what might be right."

She felt she was starting life all over again. The extra weight she had gained – 30 pounds – put pressure on her knees. It was often painful to walk up stairs. She knew that losing the extra weight and building strength was the first best step to finding her own identity.

Six months after Jim died, Pam's daughter gave her a

present of training with me. "I needed the guidance, discipline, and the structure to get my life together – to learn to take charge of myself," said Pam, almost 60 at the time. Since she really hadn't focused on herself for so long, she wasn't sure what kinds of goals would be fun and yet reasonable. An objective perspective from another person, she thought, would increase the chances of success and weekly check-ins with someone following her progress would help her commit and be accountable. Being uncertain about the proper course of training, she employed me to introduce new training techniques and exercises, adjust workouts, provide articles of interest, and occasionally just to cheer, push, or empathize with whatever happened during the previous week. "It was my first experience of focusing on myself," she said. "And it opened up a whole new world."

Setting an athletic goal did not come naturally to Pam. "I was not athletic. I was not competitive. I never had been, never will be. Don't want to be. I learned in elementary school that I do not have sufficient eye hand coordination to play sports. I was always last to be chosen for any team. Physical education requirements in college confirmed the above, so I sailed through adulthood blissfully unconcerned with exercise of any kind other than daily running around after kids, errands, housework, and gardening." But now, she wanted to lose weight and, what the heck, try something new: an athletic goal and the *MOVE!* method.

First, she set a six-week physical goal that included cross country skiing on a Nordic track, weight training with three pound weights, and stretching. Every six weeks she set another, slightly more demanding short-term goal.

"I learned to set small, achievable goals and work up to bigger and better things slowly – but surely." Within three years she had lost the 30 pounds, she was running regularly and she successfully hiked Mount Monadnock in New Hampshire. She joined a trekking trip in the Laurentian Mountains and then returned there six months later for a snowshoeing trip. "I never would have dreamed I could do any of this – and not only survive but also enjoy these events," she said.

She recalled a snowshoeing experience in the Laurentians that built her confidence in risking and achieving goals in other areas of life. "My biggest fear was of falling," she said. "There I was on snowshoes on a narrow, icy mountain trail. Solid footing? There was none. There was a tree in the way of the path. Trying to get around the tree, my feet went out from under me. I slid half way down the hill at the bottom of which was a fast moving stream. Fortunately I got hung up on the only sapling in sight. That little thing saved me.

"After discovering that I was still both alive and unhurt, I had to figure out how to get up the icy hill with snowshoes and poles all together. Fortunately I had coaching from the others up on the trail, many of whom were equally fearful of being in the same jam I was. I was finally rescued by a macho Frenchman who somehow walked down the hill and hauled me up by my armpits -- at which point I sat on the trail, waited for my breath to return and the blood to clear from my flaming cheeks. Then I just got back up and got on with it."

The physical confidence she gained helped her reevaluate other aspects of her life and address more emotionally charged issues. "Achieving physical goals helps you take charge of all aspects of life," she said. "Going for a physical goal gives you something you can control. Ultimately the only thing you can control is yourself – what you do, what you think, how you feel. You're the only person who can do that, and it's very much worth doing. I lost the weight. I got strong and I found myself.

"Learning to take risks that I never before dreamed I might take, led me to discover things that I was good at and things that I liked. When you gain some mastery over yourself, then you develop the confidence to reach out to others. Your whole world opens up, and you can find a meaningful place in it."

She took risks and made changes in other areas of life. Using concepts of the *MOVE!* method, she redesigned her house. "I decided I wanted to stay in our house of 34 years and fix everything that was wrong with it. I cleared out the clutter, opened up the space and brought in the light," she said. "That became symbolic of my whole life."

She began attending social functions with confidence on her own. A supporter of the Metropolitan Opera, she often attended dinners before concerts with other members. "When you've been part of a couple for decades, it can be hard to enter new social situations where you don't know anyone. The first time at a dinner, I was seated at a table with people whom I had never met before and I just felt uncomfortable and terribly insecure."

But the social insecurity didn't last. Her experience with the hiking and trekking groups built her confidence to hold her own anywhere. "Going into a group of people I didn't know helped me learn that it's OK to stand alone. You don't have to put on an act or talk if you don't feel like it. I remember telling myself 'I can do this too.'"

She gained the confidence to travel alone internationally. "I can go any place now. I had never done it before, but my passport is now full. I even managed to survive getting lost in the St. Petersburg Airport in Russia – and stay calm. My physical experiences of 'feel the fear and do it anyway' helped."

The process of identifying her own athletic goals ultimately helped Pam identify and realize a new mission in life: to help other families dealing with Alzheimer's. "I realized I had the ability to convey our experience, which was often far more positive than usual, and to help them find their own way more meaningfully through the journey," she said. Pam began volunteering regularly at the Alzheimer's Association counseling others on the "Help Line," a phone-in support system. She began teaching workshops, and leading support groups. "Patients and caregivers are both equally vulnerable," she said. "The struggle is hard but it need not be destructive or without hope. People can live full, productive, and valuable lives even in the face of such grave difficulties. Help is available; the trick is to learn where to find it and how to use it. That message is a distillation of my experience and my beliefs."

Pam subsequently served on the Massachusetts Board of the Alzheimers Association for six years and, as of this writing, is a member of the Leadership Council. She has also served on several Board Committees. "I often found that my voice was the strongest and sometimes the only voice for the Association's education and support programs, which are every bit as fundamental as talking about fund raising, research, and advocacy." In 2009, she won the Person of the Year award from the Massachusetts/New Hampshire Chapter of the Alzheimer's Association.

"Like my physical goals, my involvement with the Alzheimers Association developed by taking one step at a time, with the vision of what could be and the goal to help others achieve the best outcome possible. Today I am happy. I'm on my own. I am happy at home with my little dog. Exercising is an integral part of my life, as is eating little and well. I've realized that if you don't risk failing or even making a fool of yourself, you can't accomplish anything. If you fail, it's not the end of the world. Others are always there to help. You pick yourself up and go on. When the next person fails, you pick them up.

"One does not need to be an athlete or competitive to benefit immensely from physical training. The training must be physical, because it is through physical exertion that one can acquire self knowledge, self confidence, strength, perseverance, patience with oneself and the assurance that one can always start over, and one can always start again – step by step, one step at a time…in everything you do." That is the essence of *MOVE!*.

Taking On A Leadership Position

You've met Cheryl Suchors already. She's the hiker who climbed the 48 4,000-Footers in New Hampshire. Recalling what drew her to *MOVE!* in the first place, Cheryl explained that her mother had just died and she wanted guidance and support. "I was really grieving. I was so sad and I just thought that if I worked with someone who gave me a goal, it would be like having someone care about what was going on my daily life like my mother did. I thought it would be a good idea to get in shape. It was to get me out of my head."

Like Pam, Cheryl found that achieving physical goals with the *MOVE!* method affected her role in the larger world. In hiking the 48 mountains, Cheryl learned a number of critical skills that she eventually applied in the world of politics. Goal setting, recruiting, coordinating and managing people, and teaching – all skills she refined while hiking – she applied to her work in politics, as well.

"Forty-eight mountains are a lot of mountains and I needed a pool of people I could draw from to go with me. I always had to find new hiking buddies." Often her recruiting efforts involved considerable persuasion – as well as evaluating

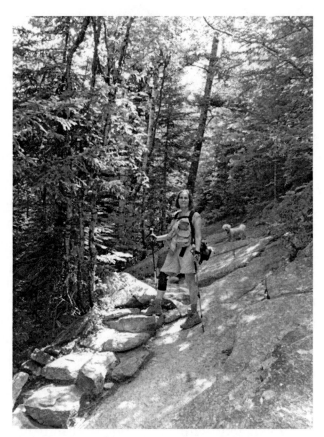

Cheryl Suchors hiking up Mount Chocorua
with her dog, Juniper.

others. "I talked about hiking to everyone I knew. I had to make it interesting to people. I had to assess whether they were fit enough and committed enough to do this." She did not know some of the people very well, and needed to decide whether they'd fit with her style of hiking. "There are ways that I like to hike and ways that I don't like to hike, so for each person joining me, it wasn't just a question of fitness but of fit. Would they be interested in looking at wild flowers or animals? Or were they only interested in going as fast as they could go?"

Coordinating and managing other hikers was just as challenging at times as recruiting them. Reviewing maps and selecting trails as well as organizing schedules – including logistics about meeting places for as many as seven or eight hikers – called for a leader. Cheryl reveled in the role. Often, as on her "mother-daughter" hike, the hikers were quite disparate. "The daughters were 15 to 18 years old and the mothers from mid- to late-fifties," she said. "There were three mothers, three daughters, and a mother without a daughter. The daughters sprinted up like rabbits but one mother, in particular, hiked quite slowly. The difference in speed became an issue when it was cold and wet."

Leading hikers, Cheryl found herself educating others about everything from food and equipment, to making decisions about weather, to when they would take breaks and how to handle the unexpected. "I did a lot of training on my hikes, she said, "but I did a lot of learning, too." Eventually Cheryl began taking leadership courses at the Appalachian Mountain Club. Courses in wilderness first aid and medical emergencies as well as the AMC protocol for leading hikes qualified her to lead the club's trips.

Goal setting, recruiting, coordinating and managing people, and teaching, were all skills she drew upon when Hillary Clinton announced her candidacy for President. Cheryl was ready to take action. "When Clinton announced, I had a Team Hillary organizing meeting at my house in October of 2007. I wound up dedicating the next eight months to Senator Clinton's campaign to become the first woman President." Cheryl took on local and cross-state leadership roles in the campaign.

Her involvement with the Hillary campaign spurred Cheryl on to continue her activist role regarding feminist issues. She created her own website on which she posts blogs about all her passions: the status of women in the world, politics, hiking, nature, and writing.

"I realize that I have become a more public person. I speak out about my position on issues to help gather other people to my causes," said Cheryl.

Doing Good By Doing Well

Antonia started working with me in her late thirties, wanting more direction in her life overall. "I felt I was floundering," said the mother of two, a former investment banker and squash player. She was a natural for the *MOVE!* method. "I was drawn to a structure of setting a goal and breaking it down into weekly tasks and having a plan for each day. A big goal that you can break into parts keeps you from being overwhelmed. A goal helps you get stuff done in your life. You feel life is moving forward."

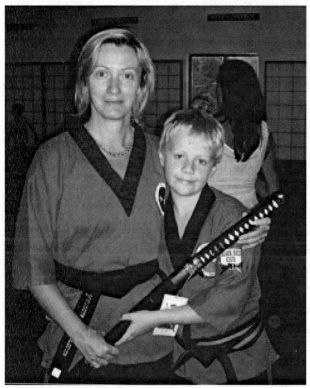

Antonia being awarded her black belt, with son Theo.

Her goals included lowering her times in middle distance races and completing her black belt in Tae Kwon Do.

Antonia Hieronymus looks back on her achievement of earning a black belt as a source of inspiration when she thinks about another goal and challenge: to collect money from her town in Massachusetts to build a school in Peru. "I have embarked on a project to involve my entire town - from schoolchildren to the senior center, from churches and temples to retail businesses and banks - to come together as a community and for each town resident to collect money, even if it's only coins, for a week in February," she said.

The goal is to collect $10,000 to build a school in Atuen, Peru. "The opportunities of the project are twofold. Firstly, it will bring my community together and strengthen our ties to one another, and secondly it will significantly impact the lives of an entire community. The challenge is clearly great. "Who am I, a suburban housewife, to accomplish this? Well, now I am someone who achieves goals."

She acknowledges that this effort, like her effort to achieve a black belt in Tae Kwon Do, will throw her into the "no-comfort" zone. Remembering her journey towards a black belt, she is confident that she can achieve this new goal as well. "Four years ago, I was a stay-at-home mum with a part-time job as a photographer, happy in my little world. Earning a black belt was a lofty goal which required me to learn some new skills....I needed to dream big. I needed to test my courage and overcome fears.

"My fledgling belief in myself was, at first small, in the face of the chorus of nay-saying doubts. They don't hand out black belts on street corners because they are difficult to come by and represent something quite special," she said. "To reach my goal I needed to prioritize my training, which sounds simple to write, but is difficult to execute. I had to say 'no' to family and clients, constantly rearrange my schedule to accommodate the extra work, and cope with the frustration of friends and family about my lack of availability and the guilt that accompanied that. As I progressed on my quest, my family started to admire my dedication and switched to being supportive of my endeavor.

"I needed to be resolute when training," she said. "I learned to weather the storms of uncertainty and feelings of wanting to quit because it wasn't worth it, both of which were really due to self-doubt. At first I didn't really want to talk enthusiastically about my black belt quest, both because I felt foolish and childish when waxing lyrical about it, and because I feared looking yet more foolish if I failed. Over the following months I learned that speaking positively about my objective reinforced it."

After four years, Antonia earned her black belt. "I wear it with pride not only because of its beautiful embroidered Korean symbols of strength and power but also because of how it reminds me of my journey," she said. "I am beginning to feel unstoppable in achieving any objective I take on in the future.

"Of course, there are many road blocks and problems in any project and my old doubts and laziness creep in at the door at every turn, but my experience of dreaming big, being dedicated, and being resolute allow me to overcome the problems."

So far, Antonia has collected $14,000, and "the money's still coming."

Conclusion

*"We are what we repeatedly do.
Excellence then is not an act but a habit."*
- Aristotle

MOVE! takes you on a journey and helps you get more out of life.

MOVE! develops your identity not only in athletics but also in all areas of life.

Find inspiration from more and more older women who are going for it.

Why wait to MOVE!?

Achieving goals can be mystifying and frustrating without the proper techniques to reach the finish line. Just the word "goal" is challenging and charged. We tend to focus just on setting goals, not on preparing for, managing, assessing, and modifying them. The fact is, with everything else going on in life, commitments are difficult to sustain and goals are hard to achieve without writing them down, without support, and without a coach. *MOVE!* helps you set your ladder against the "right" wall and climb to the top, achieving your goal and giving you a wonderful sense of accomplishment. It makes you excited to take on your next goal.

MOVE! leads to the achievement of athletic goals and further developing your identity – not only in sports but beyond into other areas of your life: to family, friendships, careers, and our larger communities. Sometimes we are conscious of the effects; at other times we don't realize the benefits received until we've moved on.

Pursuing athletic goals gives you a chance to define yourself, measure success in your own terms, and – last but not least – *have fun*. Every time you take on an athletic goal you begin a journey and create an experience. Becoming absorbed in it, you change during the process. It is likely there will be moments you actually grab peak experiences of transcendence, total immersion. In the poem "Among School Children", William Butler Yeats described that feeling of immersion as well as anyone through the experience of a dancer:

"Oh body swayed to music,

O brightening glance,

How can we know the dancer from the dance?"

In the end, there's no separating you from your athletic goal. When I mentioned the quote to several women who shared their stories in this book, they understood. Their athletic goals did transform them in one way or another and, at times, there was – yes, there *was* – a feeling of elation, even magic.

That kind of transformation is there for you to experience and the *MOVE!* method is a simple, straightforward, and effective way to access it. Again, many of us set goals we don't or can't achieve which is often destructive to our overall confidence, so it's helpful to remember the five practical steps of the *MOVE!* method (goal setting is just one step of the five) and five guidelines to keep in mind as you pursue your goals:

The five practical steps that help ensure success are:

1. Prepare for goals,
2. Set goals,
3. Manage the process,
4. Assess your achievement , and
5. Set the next goal.

The five underlying guidelines are:

1. See the big picture,
2. Enter the "beginner's mind",
3. Find support,
4. Focus your practice, and
5. Remember mastery takes time.

The vision statement, forms, and training journals all reinforce the steps. Acknowledge your doubts and fears, dispel them, and move forward. Expect and accommodate some setbacks but, most importantly, accept that you are never too old to set a goal, test your strength, and amaze yourself.

So many of us can feel that our best athletic days – or our chance to become an athlete – have long gone. But who isn't curious to test one's potential to perform physically while getting older? Whether or not you've been any kind of athlete, the future is yours to build and test your endurance, speed, strength, and flexibility at any age.

Remember the telomeres – the ends of chromosomes, the structures that carry genes which scientists believe are the cell's biological clocks that impact aging? They become longer in those who exercise more. And, exercise, particularly exercise with endurance and some intensity, builds mitochondria – the "powerhouse" organelles in cells – and keeps them healthy.

And then there is Olga Kotelko. She's is an exceptional example, but the older women now excelling in athletics represent a revolution in sports. More than ever, older women athletes are role models for younger women wanting to challenge themselves. As coach for the Liberty Athletic Club, and the website coach for www.women-running-together.com, I see young women in their twenties and thirties – women who were college and elite athletes – consistently inspired not just by looking back at younger women but looking at older women who are "going" for it as well.

Mary Harada, 76, President of the Liberty Athletic Club for the past ten years, is one of those role models (though she doesn't think of herself as one). She inspires younger women from their twenties to sixties. Mary, who started running in her 30s, has run and competed through the decades. A mother of two and a professor of history during her working life, she has run her most competitive races since retiring – and it's not because there are fewer competitors in her age group. Her results over the past years are, on an age-adjusted basis, better today than her efforts three decades ago.

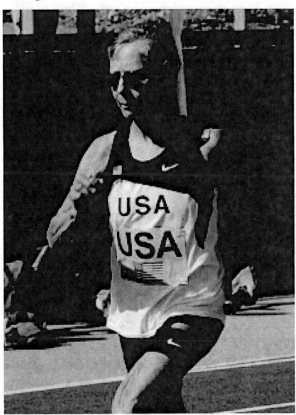

Mary Harada running in a relay at the
World Masters Athletic Championships.
PHOTOGRAPH BY TOM PHILIPS

Masters runner Carmel Papworth-Barnum – a bronze medalist in the 5 kilometer race at the 2005 World Masters Athletics Championships – described the inspiration Mary gives her: "As a woman in her mid forties I am so happy to have an athlete like Mary Harada on the running scene. In our youth obsessed culture there is so much negativity about getting older," she said. "However, women like Mary prove that you can still strive to be your best at any age. Watching her inspires me to keep running, stay healthy and, I hope, compete in my 70s and beyond. Mary clearly enjoys her running and the friendships it brings and we can aspire to that."

Regardless of your age and regardless of your experience, *MOVE!* can help you achieve the athletic or, as we've seen, non-athletic goal of your own design that can deliver a sense of triumph you'll always remember. Why not create and seize the journey and that feeling and moment of triumph?

MOVE!...

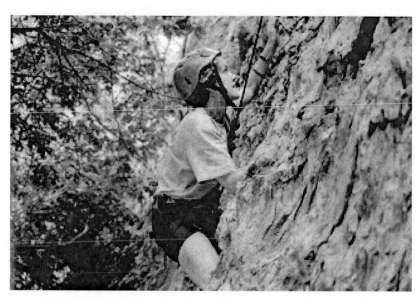

...there's nowhere to go but up!

MOVE!

Appendix

Blank Forms

1) Athletic Options
2) Big Picture Calendar
3) Vision Statement
4) Short-Term Athletic Goal
5) Weekly Self Check-In
6) Buddy Discussion
7) Weekly Training Journal
8) Short-Term Goal Review
9) Annual Athletic Goal
10) Three Month Training Calendar
11) Overcoming Doubts and Fears
12) Post-Goal Analysis, and
13) Annual Goal Review.

Athletic Options

1. List the various athletic or other activities you are considering:

     A. _____

     B. _____

     C. _____

     D. _____

2. Number of hours per week, including travel time, for your sport given other life commitments (family, household, work, community, etc.) _____

3. Specify hours you can exercise each day, including travel time:

Mon: _____ Tues: _____ Weds: _____ Thurs: _____
Fri: _____ Sat: _____ Sun: _____

4. What do you want from a sport (note top, middle, and bottom priority with a 1, 2, and 3 respectively)?

Cardiovascular fitness _____ Strength _____ Skill _____ Friendship ___
Mental challenge _____ Competitive achievement _____ Weight loss __
Decreased stress _____ Cessation of bad habits (smoking, overeating, etc.) _____ Stronger relationship with partner _____

5. List the pros and cons of each sport or activity option:

Sport: _____

Pros: _____

Cons: _____

"It is better to look ahead and prepare than to look back and regret" -Jackie Joyner Kersee

Athletic Options

Sport: _____

Pros: _____

Cons: _____

Sport: _____

Pros: _____

Cons: _____

Sport: _____

Pros: _____

Cons: _____

6. Special logistics to consider for each sport:

Outside care: _____

Pet care: _____

Equipment needed: _____

Coach available: _____

Place to train needed: _____

Others to train with: _____

Hours of travel required: _____

"It is better to look ahead and prepare than to look back and regret" -Jackie Joyner Kersee

Athletic Options (cont.)

7. Based on the pros and cons above, what's it going to be?

_____

8. Consult with a doctor about your choice.

9. Make a commitment to try your sport on a particular day and "try it" three times.

"It is better to look ahead and prepare than to look back and regret" -Jackie Joyner Kersee

Big Picture Calendar

Responsibilities	January	February	March	April	May	June
Family/ Friends						
Personal						
Work						
Home						
Athletic						

"Just go out there and do what you've got to do." -Martina Navratilova

Big Picture Calendar (cont.)

Responsibilities	July	August	September	October	November	December
Family/ Friends						
Personal						
Work						
Home						
Athletic						

"Just go out there and do what you've got to do." -Martina Navratilova

Big Picture Calendar

1. What is my long-term goal?

2. How will the commitments listed above affect my pursuit of that goal?

3. How will I handle "distractions" so they're compatible with my life as a whole?

"Just go out there and do what you've got to do." -Martina Navratilova

Vision Statement

Dream it. Speak it. Write it. Believe it.

Type and frame your vision statement to make it real and permanent. Short, concise statements are more effective than long ones because they are easier to remember (two sentences at most). Put it in a place (bedside table or other) where you can see and think about it every day.

Athletes have vision. *What's yours?*

------------------------------------CUT HERE--

My vision: _____

_____

_____

"Perseverance is failing nineteen times and succeeding the twentieth." - Julie Andrews

Short-Term Athletic Goal

Goal: _____

Current level: _____

Beginning Date: _____

Ending Date: _____

# of weeks: _____

Process Goals (Identify times per week)

Cardiovascular training: _____

_____

Intensity: _____

Strength: _____

Flexibility: _____

Mental (reading, meditations, vision statements, etc.): _____

_____

Skill development: _____

Nutrition: _____

Other (Balance, coordination): _____

"We can do anything we want as long as we stick to it long enough." - Helen Keller

Short-Term Athletic Goal (cont.)

Challenges ahead:

1. _____

2. _____

3. _____

4. _____

5. _____

NON-ATHLETIC GOALS

1. _____

2. _____

3. _____

OPTIONS FOR BUDDY

1. _____

2. _____

3. _____

"We can do anything we want as long as we stick to it long enough." - Helen Keller

Weekly Self Check-In

Date: _____

Week # : _____

Have you written down what you did in the simplest terms?

What was the plan for the past week and did you follow it?

What is the plan for this week?

If you got sick or encountered another obstacle, do you need to adjust your goal date?

How is your energy?

If you are not doing enough, what is holding you back? Are you doing too much? Have you been too ambitious? Should you consider scaling back your overall goal or adjust the time estimated to achieve it? Can you adjust the smaller goals leaving the long-term goal intact?

"You can't win them all -- but you can try." -Babe Didrikson

Buddy Discussion

Topics for discussions/issues regarding Short-Term Goal Form and
Training Journal:

1. Are your goals still realistic given your other commitments?
2. What are your greatest fears (hot weather, doubts, etc.)?
3. How can you overcome those fears?
4. Discuss training records and your weekly training journal.
5. Other.

Discuss and record solutions to your issues.

1. _____

_____

2. _____

_____

3. _____

_____

Action Plan:

_____

_____

_____

_____

_____

_____

_____

"No one changes the world who isn't obsessed." -Billie Jean King

Weekly Training Journal

Weekly Training	
Short-term physical goal:	
Start Date:	
Finish Date:	
RECORD FOR WEEK # _____ Goals for week?	
Monday	
Tuesday	
Wednesday	
Thursday	
Friday	
Saturday	
Sunday	

Not accomplished in weekly goal:

_____

"God gives talent. Work transforms talent into genius." –Anna Pavlova

Short-Term Goal Review

Beginning Date: _____
Ending Date: _____

Did you reach your goal? Yes _____ No _____

Rate your performance on the following applicable components on a scale of 1 to 5, with 1 representing weakest and 5 representing greatest effort:

Cardiovascular training: _____
Intensity: _____
Strength: _____
Flexibility: _____
Mental (reading, meditations, vision statements, etc.): _____
Skill development: _____
Nutrition: _____
Other (balance, coordination): _____

Challenges overcome:

1. _____

2. _____

3. _____

4. _____

5. _____

"Champions keep playing until they get it right." -Billie King

Short-Term Goal Review

What have you learned in this process?

1. _____

2. _____

3. _____

4. _____

5. _____

Are other commitments being met?

"Champions keep playing until they get it right." -Billie King

Annual Athletic Goals

Beginning Date: _____
Ending Date: _____

1. _____

2. _____

3. _____

4. _____

5. _____

OTHER COMMITMENTS:

1. _____

2. _____

3. _____

4. _____

5. _____

"Racing teaches us to challenge ourselves. It teaches us to push beyond where we thought we could go." -Patti Sue Plummer

Three Month Training Plan

Year: _____ Month: _____

Monday	Tuesday	Wednesday	Thursday	Friday	Saturday	Sunday	Week Totals

"True champions aren't always the ones that win, but those with the most guts." -Mia Hamm

Three Month Training Plan (cont.)

Year: _____ Month: _____

Monday	Tuesday	Wednesday	Thursday	Friday	Saturday	Sunday	Week Totals

"True champions aren't always the ones that win, but those with the most guts." -Mia Hamm

Three Month Training Plan (cont.)

Year: _____   Month: _____

Monday	Tuesday	Wednesday	Thursday	Friday	Saturday	Sunday	Week Totals

"True champions aren't always the ones that win, but those with the most guts." Mia Hamm

Overcoming Doubts and Fears

Given your goal, what is a major hurdle or fear that could harm your enjoyment and performance? (If you face hurdles, you may complete this form several times.)

> Can you identify a technique – mental, physical, or logistical – that will help you deal with the hurdle?

1. _____

2. _____

3. _____

4. _____

5. _____

6. _____

7. _____

8. _____

9. _____

10. _____

Statement that you will overcome that doubt or fear:

_____

_____

"No matter how far life pushes you down, no matter how much you hurt, you can always bounce back." -Sheryl Swoopes

Post-Goal Analysis

Event: _____

1. What was your goal? _____

2. What was you actual result? _____

3. What were your hopes? _____

4. What were your fears? _____

5. On a scale of 1 to 10 with 10 representing "Most" and "1" representing "Least", how would you rate your....

     Physical readiness -- _____

     Mental readiness -- _____

6. Comments on any particular circumstances to note related to the day of the event (logistics, weather, etc.)?

"When I go out on the ice, I just think about my skating. I forget it is a competition."
-Katarina Witt

Post-Goal Analysis (cont.)

7. Summarize your weekly physical and mental training over the past 3 months (duration, intensity, frequency of workouts – drills, etc.)

Physical Training and Mental Training (Review of Weekly Training Journal):

Weekly routine, 3 months (weeks 8 – 12) before the goal:

Weekly routine, 2 months (weeks 4 – 7) before the goal:

Weekly routine, 1 month (weeks 0 – 4) before the goal:

"When I go out on the ice, I just think about my skating. I forget it is a competition."
-Katarina Witt

Post-Goal Analysis (cont.)

8. What other life events (related to work, personal life, events of the day etc.) affected – helped or hindered – your training over the past 3 months?

9. If you attempt that same or another goal, how would you improve your training?

Other Comments:

"When I go out on the ice, I just think about my skating. I forget it is a competition."
-Katarina Witt

Annual Goal Review

Beginning Date: _____
Ending Date: _____

1. _____

2. _____

3. _____

4. _____

5. _____

SURPRISE MILESTONES

1. _____

2. _____

OTHER COMMITMENTS

1. _____

2. _____

3. _____

4. _____

5. _____

"Hard work has made it easy. That is my secret. That is why I win." -Nadia Comaneci

APPENDIX

All blank forms
are also available on
www.movegoals.com.

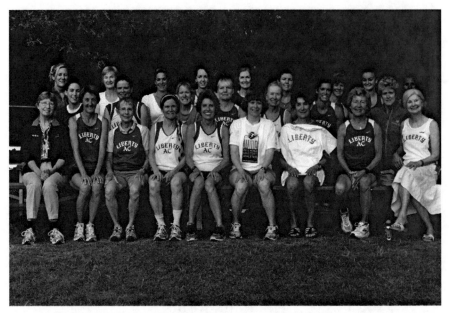

*Liberty Athletic Club age group records and championships,
2006 to present:*

*- 3 world and 4 American age group records
- 3 world age group gold medals and
- 30 national masters age group championships (track and field, cross
country, and road races).*

*Back Row, Left to Right: Janet Berg, Carrie Parsi, Leslie Ouellette,
Pam Linov, Karen Shanley, Denise Nolan, Annmarie O'Brien, Shayna
Linov, Leslie Cooper Golemme*

*Middle Row, Left to Right: Jennifer Daigle, Bethany Edwards, Beth
Soukhanov, Kelly Keelan, Regina Wright, Kristen Allen, me*

*Front Row, Left to Right: Chris Anderson, Dru Pratt-Otto, Mary Ha-
rada, Sue Gustafson, Leni Webber, Karen Lein, Molly Johnson, Marcia
Puryear, Sandy Hayes*

About the Author

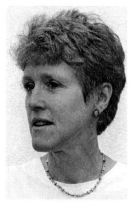

Catharine Utzschneider has focused her personal and professional interests on achieving athletic goals for fulfillment and life balance. Dr. Utzschneider earned a B.A. from Middlebury College and an M.B.A. and Ed.D. (human movement) from Boston University. There she wrote her doctoral dissertation comparing national- and world-class masters runners who starting running when young with those who started running after 30. For the past 20 years, she has run a coaching practice using the *MOVE!* method. Since 2006, she has taught goal setting and competitive performance at Boston College. She consults with athletic and educational organizations and corporations about goal setting and the *MOVE!* method.

Cathy began running competitively at 40. She became a member of the Liberty Athletic Club and for three years served as its president, securing club sponsorship from New Balance. Between 40 and 50, she achieved a #5 in the world age group ranking, and won 5 USA Track and Field age-group titles as well as a silver medal at the Nike World Masters Games. In 2010, she and Liberty teammates set an American age group record in the 4 X 1600 meter relay.

Cathy has been head coach of the Liberty Athletic Club since 2006 . She is a certified USA Track and Field coach, a certified practitioner in the Burdenko water training method, a website coach and blogger for www.women-running-together.com, and a columnist for National Masters News. Cathy is married and has two children.

www.movegoals.com

Index

Kunkemueller, Pam, 124–125, 212–216

lacrosse, 58, 90–91
leadership skills, from achieving goals, 211, 215, 217–218
Lehane, Lesley, *22*
Lein, Karen, *254*
Levy, Allan, 147
Liberty Athletic Club, 21, 192, 193, 225–226, 254, *254*
Linov, Pam, *254*
Linov, Shayna, *254*
logbooks. *See* journals, training logs
logistical support, 30, 72, 74
Loneliness (Cacioppo), 72
longevity, exercise and, 27–28
Lopez, Milena, 37

Malloy, Joe, *43*, 44
Marianne T., 182–185
Mars, Shelly, 76, *76*
martial arts, 56, 128
Martin, Kathy, 129–130, *129*
Massachusetts Board, Alzheimer's Association, 215
mastery, achieving, 36, 57, 62, 67, 76–79, 173, 214, 225
McConnell, Betsy, 36–37, 42
medical conditions, and pursuing athletic goals, 126–128
meditation, 174–175
mentoring, 177, 196. *See also* coaches, coaching
milestones, surprise, 166–167
Milford Daily (newspaper), 193
Miller, Karin, 54–56, 128
mind-body connection, 57
mistakes, allowing for, 71–82
mitochondria, 39–40
moderation, importance of, 141, 143–144

Morse, Jane, 92–93, 131
motivation. *See also* buddy system; coaches, coaching
adults' need for, 44–45
and athletic goals, 41–42
athletic goals vs. fitness routine, 35
and need for support, 37, 72
mountain climbing, 53
MOVE! method. *See also* doubts, overcoming; fears, overcoming; goals, athletic; goal setting; setbacks
broad applicability of, 20, 29, 43–44, 48–50, 57, 223–224
development of, history, 29–31
effectiveness, 31, 62–63
guidelines, underlying, 57, 62, 225
overview, 25, 26, 29, 58–60
as practical approach, 19, 57, 224
Mulroy, Kathleen, 135
muscle volume, 28, 40, 128

Navratilova, Martina, 47, 97, 98, 99, 233, 234, 235
"neutral zone," 204–205
"no comfort" zone, 67, 71
Nolan, Denise, *254*
nonagenarians, athletic competition among, 28
nutrition, 90, 108, 149

O'Brien, Annmarie, 69–70, *254*
Olympic Triathlon Team, 44
Ouellette, Leslie, 89–90, *89*, *254*
outcome goals, 95, 107
Overcoming Doubts and Fears form, 123, 136, 138–139, 248
overweight or obese bodies, 51, 100, 124, 136, 212
Overwhelmed: Coping with Life's

CPSIA information can be obtained at www.ICGtesting.com
Printed in the USA
LVOW111651110512

281384LV00011B/84/P